CONJURING SCIENCE

5·28·97

CONJURING SCIENCE

■ ■ ■ ■ ■ ■ ■ ■ ■ ■ ■ ■ ■ ■ ■ ■ ■ ■ ■

*Scientific Symbols
and Cultural Meanings
in American Life*

■ ■ ■ ■ ■ ■ ■ ■ ■ ■ ■ ■ ■ ■ ■ ■ ■ ■ ■

Christopher P. Toumey

RUTGERS UNIVERSITY PRESS
New Brunswick, New Jersey

Library of Congress Cataloging-in-Publication Data

Toumey, Christopher P., 1949–
        Conjuring science : scientific symbols and cultural meanings in
        American life / Christopher P. Toumey.
                p. cm.
        Includes bibliographical references and index.
        ISBN 0-8135-2284-6 (cloth : alk. paper). — ISBN 0-8135-2285-4
        (pbk. : alk. paper)
                1. Science—Social aspects—United States.   2. Ethnology—United
        States.   3. Anthropology—United States.   4. Symbolism.   I. Title.
        Q175.5.T68   1996
        306.4'5'0973—dc20   95-43282
                                                                                                CIP

British Cataloging-in-Publication information available

To Eileen Toumey London,
the best mother a writer could have

CONTENTS

■ ■ ■

ACKNOWLEDGMENTS

■ ■ ■

I am grateful to many people for contributions, tangible and intangible, to this book. First and foremost I thank my best friend, Kathryn Luchok, for much sensible advice, many delightful conversations, and for all the kinds of love that make me glad I married her. Next is David Hess, whose constructive criticisms of my manuscript helped me improve this book greatly.

My students made me refine my thinking when they held me to high standards of teaching. In particular I have in mind those students in my seminars on Science, Technology and Human Values at Duke University, those students in my anthropology courses at the University of North Carolina, and my student-inmates at Central Prison in Raleigh.

Elizabeth Jones engaged me in a series of excellent conversations in 1992 about the theoretical basis of the anthropology of science. Carole Crumley, Gary Downey, Ray Eve, Les Harrison, Will Kimler, Tom McIver, Ronald Numbers, William Pollitzer, Eric Poncelet, George Webb, the late George Holcomb, and other friends encouraged me and appreciated my writing, thereby lifting me from the misery of academic invisibility.

The family Magallanes—Fernando, Ronna, Paloma, Gabriela, and Maximiliano—wanted me to be intellectual but let me be silly. The Department of Anthropology at the University of North Carolina and the Program in Science, Technology and Human Values at Duke University each gave me honest work, with no heavy lifting, during the early days of writing this book. Martha Heller, Karen Reeds, and other good friends at Rutgers University Press wrapped my writing in the finest of professional care.

I also want to say a word about Connie Jenkins, Kenneth Foon, and Patrick McGrath, who are my favorite family doctor, my favorite oncologist, and my favorite surgeon, respectively. When I was ill, they offered me a great deal. If I would relinquish my spleen, I would recover my health. They kept the bargain, and I think they're great.

In addition, the *Journal of the American Academy of Religion* and *Science, Technology & Human Values* published longer versions of Chapters Eight and Nine, in 1993 and 1992 respectively, for which I am grateful. I would also like to thank *Public Understanding of Science* for publishing a version of Chapter Seven in 1996.

■ ■ ■

A note on words and meanings: I freely use adjectives and nouns like "American" and "Americans" to refer to the culture and the people of the United States. I understand that many of the peoples of the Western Hemisphere consider themselves Americans in the geographical sense that their homes are in North America or South America and that they resent it when the geographical meaning is reduced to the national meaning (referring only to the United States), thereby making many millions of Americans un-American, so to speak. Some writers solve this problem by dropping the national usage entirely and replacing it with the adjective "U.S.," as in "U.S. Army" or "the U.S. government." That way, American *national* culture becomes "U.S. culture," the people of the fifty states become "the U.S. people," and so on. I feel that in most cases this latter usage is awkward and sometimes downright dumb. A better solution, I think, is to state candidly at the beginning of a book that the author is using American and Americans in the *national* sense only, without implying anything about the geographical identities of our American neighbors in North and South America.

PART ONE

Science and American Values

■ ■ ■

CHAPTER ONE

Science in an Old Testament Style

In 1988, a television commercial for a common drugstore product made an uncommon claim about the endorsement of medical science. An actor from a daytime soap opera appeared on-screen in a white lab coat and declared, "I'm not a doctor, but I play one on TV." Then with those credentials he endorsed the product, recommending it in the authoritative voice of a medical doctor.

Such a commercial would be preposterous if it were generally recognized that there is a real difference between a doctor with genuine credentials and an actor who plays a doctor on TV. After all, the actor who played a doctor was not a doctor, and he candidly declared that he was not.

If a real physician is a symbol of medical science once removed from that kind of abstract institutional authority, and if an actor who pretends to be a doctor, like Robert Young as Marcus Welby, M.D., is a symbol twice removed, then the actor who did not even pretend to be a doctor was thrice removed from medical science. Nevertheless, for the purpose of pitching the product, he was an effective simulacrum of the authority of medical science.

■ ■ ■

The town of Mew Madrid, Missouri, devoted itself single-mindedly to emergency preparations for an earthquake in November and December 1990. The city council stockpiled drinking water, the mayor positioned his fire trucks in open fields far from buildings that might collapse, the local elementary school canceled classes for the day the earthquake was expected to hit, and the local insurance business sold many earthquake policies. At nearby St. John Missionary Baptist

Church, Sunday school on December 2 began with the invocation to "Bless all of us, oh Father, that are upset about the earthquake."

The reason? Iben Browning, Ph.D., had predicted that a massive earthquake of at least 6.5 Richter had a 50 percent chance of striking New Madrid on December 3, 1990. It was said that Browning had predicted California's 1989 Loma Prieta earthquake. Surely an earthquake warning from someone with credentials and experience like Browning's was serious scientific advice, not to be taken lightly. Indeed, David Stewart, Ph.D., a geophysicist at nearby Southeast Missouri State University, endorsed Dr. Browning's prediction for 1990 in Missouri.

In truth, Iben Browning's Ph.D. was in zoology, not seismology. He had not predicted the Loma Prieta event. His supporter, David Stewart, had previously employed paranormal methods, including the services of psychic Clarissa Bernhardt from the *National Enquirer,* to anticipate an earthquake in North Carolina that never happened. The National Earthquake Prediction Evaluation Council, under the auspices of the U.S. Geological Survey, adamantly denounced the faulty logic of Browning's seismological theories.

No matter. Tens of thousands of people in the region around New Madrid changed their plans and their behavior in anticipation of Iben Browning's earthquake. And never mind the skeptical bureaucrats of the U.S. Geological Survey, who seemed indifferent to the worries of the people of New Madrid. Was it not better to choose concerned scientists like Iben Browning and David Stewart as one's friends and advisers?

Tension was as bad as it could be when December 3, 1990 came around. But the earth did not shake.

■ ■ ■

For many years, the tobacco lobby challenged the conclusion that smoking causes cancer, by drawing a hard distinction between the kind of scientific proof that comes from replicable demonstrations of cause and effect, and the epidemiological conclusions that are drawn from statistical correlations: the absolute proof of test-tube science, so to speak, versus the uncertainty of statistical probability. Then with scientific proof defined in terms of test-tube science, the tobacco advocates argued that scientists have not proven that smoking causes cancer since they have not elucidated the biochemical pathways by which the cause (smoking) leads to the effect (cancer). True, scientists have not, so the tobacco advocates are correct, provided that scientific proof is defined this way.

This logic implicitly compares the value of one form of scientific reasoning with that of another: a statistical conclusion is always inferior to a replicable demonstration of causation since the former is always less than 100 percent certain. More to the point, one can then say that the smoking and cancer connection is *possible* but far from certain, which is enormously useful to smokers who want a reason for not giving up smoking and to those who want to sell them tobacco products.

In June 1993, attorneys for the tobacco industry initiated a lawsuit to reverse the decision of the Environmental Protection Agency (EPA) designating secondhand smoke as a carcinogen. Their legal reasoning centered on the issue of statistical significance. Six of the thirty studies cited by the EPA had confidence levels of 95 percent ($p < .05$) for the conclusion that secondhand smoke causes cancer, but the other twenty-four studies had lower levels, for example, 80 or 85 percent.

Was this really a change in the standards of scientific proof? It seems to have been since the attorneys for the tobacco interests implicitly conceded that epidemiological-statistical methods *might* have scientific merit, provided that they met confidence levels of 95 percent or above (which is entirely reasonable for epidemiological research that has real policy implications). But the weaker studies had an equally important role in this argument. Every scientific study with a confidence level less than 95 percent could be interpreted to impeach all the studies with a level greater than 95 percent. So epidemiological-statistical studies of carcinogenicity can now be legally credible, but only in the sense that weaker studies have the effect of impeaching stronger studies, which is to say that weaker ones are more credible than stronger ones.

■ ■ ■

This medley of incidents reflects two aspects of the peculiar role of science in American culture. On the one hand, the institutional endorsement of scientific authority is so greatly respected that the TV doctor, the credentials of Iben Browning, and the august weight of test-tube scientific proof are believed to enhance the worth of drugstore products, disaster preparations, and health regulations. On the other hand, the public understanding of the scientific knowledge and scientific reasoning in which that respect is grounded is so shallow that an *appearance* of scientific authority can be easily conjured from cheap symbols and ersatz images like an actor's white lab coat, a zoologist's credentials in a controversy about seismology, and a definition of scientific proof that makes epidemiological evidence irrelevant to an epidemiological question of carcinogenicity.

In other instances, the raw material for conjuring a semblance of science might be the solemn sounds of Greek or Latin terminology, visual images of shiny laboratory paraphernalia, or graphs and charts that pop up on the monitors of humming computers. Rich and deep is the supply of scientific iconography that can be borrowed for the purpose of cobbling together an image of science.

To understand the strength of popular respect for scientific authority, consider that certain theologians speak of the plenary authority of scripture, meaning that the written word of revelation embodies all the wisdom one needs to answer any of life's questions, big or small, spiritual or secular. We can borrow the term "plenary" to describe the way many citizens feel about science. The prestige of science is so great that it, too, is believed to possess such authority and be able to answer any of life's questions. This is so because science is widely believed to transcend the social forces that obviously shape other human institutions, such as politics or religion. Science is believed to be, in a word, "objective."

Science does not really deserves such awe, nor do most scientists believe such things about it. But many nonscientists do.[1] Thus, to invoke the symbols of science is to make policies sound, commodities desirable, and behavior legitimate.[2] By definition, these things are meritorious when they have the appearance of being scientific.

And yet surrounding the plenary authority of science is a great vacuum of understanding about scientific knowledge and reasoning. Studies of science education and scientific literacy reveal that large portions of the American public do not know such essential scientific concepts as "molecule" or "radiation," cannot comprehend the methods of scientific reasoning, and could not apply either to public issues. Historical surveys of science in America demonstrate that the intangible meanings cherished within the institutional culture of science—the pleasures that make science rewarding to scientists—are alien to most of the American public.

The religion of the Old Testament could be the pattern for this combination of respect without comprehension. The chosen people believed in God, feared Him, and doubted His power only at great risk to themselves; yet they understood God very imperfectly since this being was a distant mystery who made himself known by awesome signs: burning bushes, pillars of fire, dreadful plagues. So it is with science in America today. Instead of comprehending scientific knowledge, scientific methods, or scientific standards, much of the adult population knows science only in terms of certain symbols that stand for science and that stand between people and scientific understanding. An actor who stands for medical science, for example, because he plays a doctor and wears a white lab coat, or a courtroom definition of scientific standards, or a zoologist's credentials in an argument about earthquakes.

This paradox of respect without comprehension can be broken down into three questions. First, what are the historical conditions that have caused the culture of science to be so estranged from other parts of American culture? This is a question of how science is perceived by nonscientists such that the values and meanings of science, as understood by scientists, are not well integrated into the values and meanings of American life. Scientific judgment is one thing, but nonscientists' everyday thinking about science is something else.

Second, how does science fit into American democratic culture today? Even though the values and standards of science are somewhat alien to the rest of American culture, and even though much of the American public is ill-equipped to make informed decisions about scientific issues, decisions affecting science (appropriations, legislation, policy, and the curriculum of public school science education, to name a few) are nevertheless made according to democratic processes. Science in America is strongly affected by extrascientific factors. One consequence of this effect is that various parties can invoke the symbols of science to claim that science endorses their own respective positions and can do so with little or no regard for scientific standards. Because there is too little public understanding of scientific knowledge or reasoning, it is possible to borrow, steal, distort, or manipulate these symbols for causes and ideologies that do not necessarily have anything to do with science.

That, in turn, begs the third question: if the symbols of science are being used to endorse or legitimize certain values and meanings but not the values and meanings of science, then to what exactly do these symbols refer? What do the symbols of science convey, if not the content of science? What are the nonscientific ideas that are being expressed by means of scientific symbols?

I propose to explore the conjuring of science in four parts. In part 1 (this and the next two chapters), I describe the tension between science and certain common American values. By tracing a series of changing notions about science across the last two hundred years, I suggest that science, loosely defined, fit quite comfortably into American democratic culture in the early nineteenth century. Both the empirical content and the intellectual structure of science were relatively simple, so it was easy for the average person to understand science and appreciate it. After the arrival in the United States of modern scientific thinking and methods, however, beginning around the middle of the nineteenth century, a great divergence appeared between science as understood by scientists and science as understood by other Americans.

In the gap between those two ways of understanding science, there arose a certain kind of mischief, namely, the conjuring of science. One could use the common symbols and images of science, as understood by nonscientists, to make it seem that scientists were bestowing the plenary authority of science on various causes and ideologies that had nothing to do with science. By placing this mischief in American history, we can see how and when it arose and how it has been maintained throughout the twentieth century. Also in part 1, I present two twentieth-century theories for reconciling the values of science with American democratic culture, but I conclude that both theories were badly flawed and that they failed to heal the estrangement of science from common American values.

Part 2 (chapter 4) transforms the problem of conjuring science from one of the history of science in American life to one of the anthropology of science. Undoubtedly, science occupies an important place in American life by virtue of its authority to bless or curse one commodity or another, one cause or another. But it cannot be taken for granted that the internal values and standards of science will have much effect in a public dispute about science, let alone that they will govern such a dispute. The critical question is not how science influences American culture but rather how American culture treats science. Accordingly, I first indicate one way for cultural anthropology to look at American culture. Then within that anthropological framework, I examine how the larger culture deals with science. The heart of my anthropological approach is an argument about the cultural conditions that enable various parties to separate the symbols of science from the substantive content of science so as to invoke and deploy those symbols to bestow the plenary authority of science on almost any commodity, ideology, or behavior.

Part 3 illustrates that problem by presenting five episodes of science in American life (chapters 5–9). They are "Soul-Snatching" (the case of the fluoridation controversies); "Plague" (the 1986 California referendum on acquired immunodeficiency syndrome/human immunodeficiency virus [AIDS/HIV] policy that was a Grand Guignol of scientific symbols and nonscientific meanings); "Hope" (the cold fusion controversy); "Anarchy" (the antievolutionary definition of evolution as generated by the modern creationist movement); and "Evil" (the representation of science in the mad scientist stories of fiction and film).

Lastly, part 4 (chapter 10) draws these lessons about scientific symbols and cultural meanings together into a descriptive model of science in American life.

So my argument is as follows: In American culture, science is widely believed to possess a plenary authority. But this authority is not really grounded in the values and standards of science because they are estranged from the main themes of American life. Nevertheless, symbols of science are frequently invoked to support claims that science has endorsed a given commodity or cause, which is to say that a semblance of scientific authority can be conjured. In which case, it is worth discovering what nonscientific values and meanings do the symbols of science stand for, which is a question of *why* science is conjured, and how it is that those symbols of science serve those nonscientific meanings, which is to ask *how* science is conjured.

I confess that my anthropology of science has very little to do with the methods, the knowledge, or the theories that we point to as the intellectual content of science. Instead, this anthropology is a story about how we borrow bits and pieces of science, loose and jagged, to aid our existential efforts to make sense of our lives. We think we know some things about reality or about human existence or about right and wrong, and maybe we do. But our confidence is much enhanced when we think that science endorses or corroborates the things we think we know.

Why do we think so? How do we conclude that science takes sides in moral or existential questions? Why do we believe that a policy is better if it seems that science has blessed it? Why does it appear that one person's behavior is more righteous, or another's less, when a claim is made that science recommends this habit or that?

Understand, please, that this is not an attempt to deconstruct science, as they say. In all modesty, I have little to say here about those postmodernist questions that ask whether science is real. The head-banging disputes that have set deconstructionists against positivists are not for me. I have thought much and written a little about them, but I do not let those questions derail my own ideas about how we make science a part of our common American life.

My argument is that, regardless of the metaphysical status of science, its value in American life is contingent on the cultural values and meanings that frame science. And so I offer a story not about science but about the moralities, the philosophies, the ideologies, and the beliefs that surround science. I ask how the American people attribute the plenary authority of science to those values and meanings by disconnecting the popular symbols of science from its intellectual substance and attaching those symbols to other matters instead. In other words, I ask how we conjure a semblance of science.

CHAPTER TWO

■ ■ ■

American Visions of Nature and Science

If the separation of symbols from substance appears chronic in the case of science, then we should know that it was not always like this. Science enjoyed less complicated relations of symbols to substance during the colonial and early republican years of American history. The conditions that made possible the conjuring of science arose much later. And so to understand how those latter developments came about, we need to trace the course of science in American life.

Tracing that course, however, is not as neat and final as pinning a butterfly specimen to a display board in a glass case. It is more like watching a handful of different kinds of caterpillars as they become, first, chrysalides and, later, butterflies. They vary, they wiggle, and they change. Their details are oftentimes fuzzy.

Let us begin with a generic definition: science is the systematic study of nature. Within that general statement we can find that during the past two hundred years of American history, there have been multiple understandings of what science and nature are and how they fit into our lives. Three such visions are particularly important. I call them the Protestant model, the philosophy of useful knowledge, and the European scientific research ethos. The first two constitute the prehistory to the conditions for conjuring science; the third actually generates those conditions.

THE PROTESTANT MODEL OF THE STUDY OF NATURE

During the eighteenth century and well into the nineteenth, many Protestant Americans appreciated the systematic study of nature in terms of a theology that held that God had revealed himself to us twice, in scripture and in nature. From this idea of "two revelations," it followed that curiosity about nature was a good Christian virtue, provided it was infused with the same piety that motivated one's reading of scripture. Although the methods for studying nature were different from those for scripture, the end result was expected to be the same: a Christian was morally enriched by seeing the evidence of God's character in His creation. The adaptation of a creature to its environment, for example, was a sign of God's careful design, while abundance in nature was a clue to the generosity of the Creator. Thus did the study of nature enable a person "to fathom God's plan."[1]

This model was much more than a virtuous attitude. It also included an influential threefold epistemology for aligning knowledge of nature with Protestant readings of scripture by reducing both kinds of learning to their most obvious, tangible, empirically accessible qualities. Truth, whether from nature or from scripture, was simple and was easily at hand. This way of thinking also supposed that theories and hypotheses were frivolous mental complications that interfered with the goal of grasping the truth. That last feature protected the Protestant model's simple empiricist spirit from sophisticated intellectual critiques by rendering such critiques evidence of weakness of character.[2]

The three epistemological bases of the Protestant model were the Scottish Common Sense philosophy, Baconian empiricism, and the Princeton Theology. The first of these arose in the Scottish liberal arts universities in the eighteenth century as a reaction against the specialization of knowledge. At that time many English and Continental intellectuals accepted that knowledge was rightly divided into numerous professional spheres because truth had many facets, most of which were difficult to apprehend. English and Continental thinking also presumed that nonspecialists needed the mediation of specialists to apprehend certain knowledge. The Common Sense philosophy abruptly rejected those assumptions. It proposed that things worth understanding were not particularly opaque. Rather, they were just what they appeared to be, in nature or in scripture, and a person of average intelligence could clearly see them as such. Sense perceptions were reliable, and reliable sense perceptions were common—thus, the Common Sense philosophy.[3]

When the Common Sense philosophy was applied to nature or to scripture, it placed the burden of proof on those who argued that truth was complicated and that one's perceptions had to be specialized. The strength of this position was that specialists had the impossible burden of convincing nonspecialists that only specialists could apprehend the truth. Even if, for argument's sake, the specialists' contention were true, nonspecialists still could not accept it because, by definition, they could not understand what the specialists were saying. Therefore, the logic of the Common Sense philosophy automatically discredited intellectuals who expected knowledge to be specialized, including those thinkers who expected the lessons that came from nature to be different from the lessons yielded by scripture.

Similarly, Baconian empiricism held that truth was both uncomplicated and self-evident, in which case science was a simple business of observing, collecting, and classifying the facts of nature. Theories, metaphysical thoughts, and other intellectual complications were useless.[4] In fact, they could even be *worse* than useless, in the more Puritanical reading of Baconianism: they could be evidence of a sinful attitude. The simple tasks of observing, collecting, and classifying were exercises in "the Puritan ethic of grace through work" because they were *active* chores inspired by piety.[5] Theorizing, however, was considered an idle pastime, an escape from good hard work, in which case a theory was an outward sign of an inner weakness, namely, the deadly sin of slothfulness. A pious person stayed busy by collecting and sorting specimens of plants, animals, bugs, or rocks; but an indolent person squandered time with armchair speculations about the natural world, thereby leaving himself or herself vulnerable to the kinds of mischief that fill up idle time. In this way, Baconian empiricism complemented the Scottish Common Sense philosophy by adding a harsh moral judgment to the latter's philosophy of knowledge.

Finally, the Princeton Theology (so called because it was developed at the Princeton Theological Seminary in New Jersey) applied the Common Sense philosophy and Baconian empiricism directly to the reading of scripture. In accordance with Baconian principles, this theology asserted that scripture, like nature, comprised a body of uncomplicated facts.[6] In the spirit of Common Sense, it suggested that "even simple Christians could understand the essential message of the Bible on their own."[7] The Princeton Theology was thus the keystone of the Protestant model, for it subjected knowledge of scripture to the same standards as knowledge of nature, namely, Baconian empiricism and Common Sense.

Until late in the nineteenth century, the Protestant model was the frame of reference used by most educated people to appreciate the systematic study of nature. New England Puritans had established the first free public schools. They and other Protestants had founded most of the nation's liberal arts colleges. Even at the state universities, most of the faculty were likely to have been trained in one Protestant institution or another. At all levels, the values of the curriculum were typically those of the Protestant model. This was so even in the generic term for the systematic study of nature, namely—"natural theology," which was then subdivided into "natural history" (i.e., biology and geology) and "natural philosophy" (mathematics, physics, and chemistry).

Thus it was that curiosity about nature was made quite compatible with the Protestant faith of so many citizens. It was easy for those who systematically studied nature (then called "naturalists," for there was no such term as "scientist" in the early nineteenth century) to find merit and moral enrichment in their work. Edward Hitchcock, New England preacher and geologist, typified the Protestant spirit that united scripture with nature: "Armed usually with a geologist's pick in one hand and a copy of the Bible in the other."[8]

The transmission of this particular package of values to others— other Protestants, that is—was not particularly difficult, given that curiosity about nature was simply another exercise in virtue and salvation. Anyone who could appreciate virtue and salvation could easily see the merits of the Protestant model. The substance and symbols of science were more or less the same as those of faith, which is to say that they were not particularly problematic.

THE PHILOSOPHY OF USEFUL KNOWLEDGE

A second way for nineteenth-century Americans to appreciate knowledge about the natural world was to equate it simply with engineering and technology. This way, that knowledge was nothing less than the key that would unlock the natural resources of a great continent. It would make individuals prosperous while making the masses comfortable. So, too, such knowledge would ensure that the American nation was self-sufficient and that European intellectuals were rendered impotent here. Progress, democracy, and independence—these would be the fruits of knowledge about nature.

Early American thought about natural resources and their purpose was heavily influenced by the geography of the new continent. Because these blessings were so plentiful and so ubiquitous, the small European-American population easily diffused to where the resources were, whether near the Atlantic seaboard, on the frontier, or beyond the frontier. In those circumstances, it was necessary that individuals, their families, and their small communities be highly self-sufficient. Large-scale division of labor was unthinkable. Knowledge about nature had to be nonspecialized, that is, accessible to everyone, including uneducated people. Also, it had to be useful, first for survival, later for prosperity.[9]

Thomas Jefferson, Benjamin Franklin, and a small number of other Americans embraced a different vision—namely, the European Enlightenment view of science, which subordinated useful knowledge to a larger plan of intellectual enrichment. Material increase was good, but moral progress was better, and the former was expected to serve the latter by illustrating the benefits of human reason. Historians are divided about whether the Enlightenment vision was broad or scant during Jefferson's time—and I agree with those who say scant—but truly it was all but gone by the fourth decade of the nineteenth century, eclipsed by the simple view that progress consisted of *material* increase generated from technology and uncomplicated by philosophical baggage.[10] "There was no escaping the exceedingly pragmatic view of science in the United States by 1830."[11] Indeed, "useful arts" and "mechanical arts" were the common names for this knowledge about nature, before words such as "science" and "technology" gained their current meanings.

Daniel Webster and Edward Everett were two of the main apostles for the message of useful knowledge.[12] Hugo Meier, George Daniels, and Leo Marx note that the simple materialist philosophy had its doubters and its Jeremiahs, including Thomas Carlyle, Ralph Waldo Emerson, Henry David Thoreau, Nathaniel Hawthorne, and Herman Melville, but they were a small minority until recently.[13] As the philosophy of useful knowledge unfolded in the early years of the nineteenth century, it produced four lines of reasoning about the progress that knowledge would create.

1. By making the individual prosperous, useful knowledge also made the individual free. Presumably it enabled the farmer, the mechanic, and the merchant to thrive without being either an employee or a debtor to another man.[14] For this reason, an American representative at London's Crystal Palace exhibition in 1851 described the American inventions on display as "evidence of the ingenuity, industry, and capacity of a free and educated people. . . . We showed the results of pure democracy upon the industry of men."[15] More recently, Eugene Ferguson notes that one of the democratic consequences of technology was an improvement in the social status of mechanics as a result of developments such as a "romantic . . . strain in the narrative of American involvement with its technology," and Meier describes the rise of a new form of journalism dedicated to celebrating technology as "a high and honorable calling."[16]

2. Technology improved the standard of living of the whole population by mass-producing commodities. Throughout the nineteenth century, various new technologies "were seen as providing the greatest good to the greatest number by improving transportation, enhancing communication, saving labor, and transforming the wilderness."[17] "We have universalized all the beautiful and glorious results of industry and skill," crowed Horace Greeley in 1853. "We have made them a common possession of the people. . . . We have democratized the means and appliances of a higher life."[18] When Samuel Colt stated that "there is nothing that cannot be produced by machinery," he faithfully reflected both the American optimism that progress could be mass-produced and the myopia that defined progress only in material terms.[19]

3. The fruits of useful knowledge would make the United States economically independent of foreign nations. As virtuous individuals were self-reliant, so should virtuous nations be. Or so it seemed at a time when a young nation, born of British parents and assisted by Continental midwives, fervently wanted its own unique identity, grounded in a history and economics of sui generis. Furthermore, Americans had learned that it did them no good to get entangled, willingly or not, in European misadventures such as the Napoleonic Wars. If the North American continent would supply all the necessary land, water, flora, and fauna, as seemed the case, and if useful knowledge provided the means to make good use of those resources, then Americans could blithely ignore all things European and happily pursue progress on their own.[20]

4. The spirit of useful knowledge would make the United States intellectually independent of foreign nations. It has long been a powerful theme of American thought that Old World habits are degenerate until proved otherwise; ergo, American habits ought to be antipodal to Old World habits. In Europe serious curiosity about nature had a reputation for being a rich man's hobby and richly philosophical; in the United States it had to be a working man's instrument and clearly useful. European thought was meant to yield abstract principles about nature in general; American thought had to solve tangible problems of a local quality.[21] The former was organized, stratified, sometimes centralized; the latter was much more egalitarian, or rather hopelessly decentralized, to the point that colleges and academies meant nothing to most engineers, mechanics, and inventors.

Alexis de Tocqueville's 1834 observations of Americans' unique intellectual habits are sharp, and his interpretations often brilliant. He notes that citizens of a democracy (namely, the United States) are not "naturally indifferent to science. . . . [Rather,] they cultivate [science] after their own fashion, and bring to the task their own peculiar qualifications and deficiencies."[22] These included "a taste for the tangible and the real, a contempt for tradition"; a mistrust of "visionary speculation"; an inclination "never [to be] long detained by the subtilty [*sic*] of the schools, nor ready to accept big words for sterling coin," with a preference instead for ideas expressed "in the vernacular tongue."[23]

Tocqueville gives us a fitting perspective on the merits and the faults of the American preference for useful knowledge:

> In America the purely practical part of science is admirably understood, and careful attention is paid to the theoretical portion which is immediately requisite to application. On this head the Americans always display a clear, free, original, and inventive power of mind. But scarcely anyone in the United States devotes himself to the essentially theoretical and abstract portion of human knowledge. In this respect the Americans carry to excess a tendency which is, I think, discernible, though in a less degree, among all nations. . . . Nothing is more necessary to the culture of the higher sciences, or of the more elevated departments of science, than meditation; and nothing is less suited to meditation than the structure of democratic society.[24]

The particulars of the philosophy of useful knowledge were somewhat different from those of the Protestant model, but these two visions of science and nature shared two vitally important features. First, both frameworks fitted knowledge about nature comfortably into the common American culture by making the systematic study of nature a part of a larger goodness. Second, the resulting connection between the substance of science and its symbols was therefore simple and direct. The Protestant model made natural curiosity an exercise in Christian faith, thereby yielding such symbols as the pious naturalist. The philosophy of useful knowledge connected science to prosperity, democracy, and independence, with machines, gadgets, and personal material possessions symbolizing those virtues. And so these two understandings each provided clear and simple rationales for studying the natural world, for making such methods of study an important part of Americans' lives, and for appreciating the contributions of naturalists, engineers, mechanics, and inventors.

THE EUROPEAN SCIENTIFIC RESEARCH ETHOS

A third approach to nature, barely acknowledged in America during the eighteenth and early nineteenth centuries, was the European Enlightenment model, according to which secular values, rationalist thinking, and naturalistic explanation combined to create the methods and knowledge we now call "science." Furthermore, the Enlightenment model recommended science for the sake of science, irrespective of other justifications. Thus, the merits of science were uncoupled from religious reasons, particularly the Protestant rationale for studying nature.

The Enlightenment philosophes of the eighteenth and early nineteenth centuries, including Thomas Jefferson, believed that useful knowledge and its material benefits were among the legitimate fruits of this European scientific research ethos. By the later decades of the nineteenth century, however, many of the practitioners of this scientific tradition, especially those in Germany, had devoted themselves exclusively to science for the sake of science, as if useful knowledge constituted an intellectual poison to the spirit of their work. Science in the style of the research ethos then became known as "pure," "basic," "abstract," "advanced,"or "theoretical" science, which terms are still used to name it today.

Tocqueville, when lamenting the absence of higher intellectual life in the United States, supposed that Americans could look to the English for the works of scientists, writers, and artists, and thereby "enjoy the treasures of the intellect without requiring to labour in amassing them."[25] If so, then the rise of the European scientific research ethos in this country began when the Americans of Tocqueville's day decided they should no longer subcontract their thinking to the mother country. They sought out the Enlightenment kind of science in Europe, and after they found it there, they nurtured it at home.

The first step was the experience of studying science, medicine, and engineering at European universities. Between about 1790 and 1820, Paris was the center of Europe's best scholarship in those fields. Students there ingested the habits and manners of French rationalism, particularly the notion that vast amounts of natural phenomena could be reduced to a few abstract laws, ideally in the form of mathematical equations. A scientist who was reasonably comfortable with the French structure of knowledge could then make good use of vast amounts of scientific information by combining a small number of abstract principles.

The other main European influence was the culture of experimental science in the German universities. In the German style, one could do much more than place known phenomena into natural laws; the scientist could discover many new phenomena by manipulating events in controlled conditions that imitated selected parts of nature. For this reason the German method of discovery had displaced the French approach as the most prestigious form of science well before the middle of the nineteenth century.

Far more important than the specific discoveries of the German scientists was the German academic culture that nurtured the system of discovery. Universal public education, supplemented by numerous public libraries, produced plenty of well-prepared college students. The *Lernfreiheit* (freedom to learn) gave young Germans the right to enroll in any German university and to study any subject; this right was complemented by the *Lehrfreiheit*, the professors' "freedom to teach" whatever they wanted.[26] In seminar-style courses and in specialized institutes within the universities, teaching was closely intertwined with research. A series of degrees, credentials, and academic ranks, along with prestige and rewards to suit each, offered enough career goals to fill a lifetime. This system of prestige and reward also caused scholars to match themselves against higher and higher professional standards, for instance, those of local and national scientific societies, plus those of local and national scientific journals. The various German state governments supported science through their universities and academies, but their influence was more of a gentle coordination of priorities than a strict control of resources.[27] Then (and since then) the nineteenth-century German research universities were the basic model for the institutionalization of science.[28]

Americans' experiences in the German system, combined with some indigenous American events, brought the European scientific research ethos to the United States. As the U.S. population grew, American colleges expanded. State universities of a few dozen students each quickly changed to several hundred each. Then as faculties grew proportionately, state universities shed their generalists in favor of specialists. Whereas previously one person might have taught geology, biology, and Old Testament, the newer faculty had at least one specialist in each of those fields. From this grew autonomous academic departments. When Charles Eliot pioneered the elective system at Harvard in the 1860s and 1870s, students emulated the specialization of their professors.

The Morrill Act of 1862, which established land-grant colleges, was meant to be strictly an exercise in the philosophy of useful knowledge, principally in the areas of agriculture, engineering, and military training. But the act also encouraged a European-style research ethos when schools of agriculture benefited from specialized biologists or when schools of engineering attracted specialized physicists.

The same was true of scientific work commissioned by state and national governments. Geological research, for example, which was intended only to seek out farmland, minerals, and railroad routes, inevitably also considered geological structures and their historical significance, much to the chagrin of anti-intellectual legislators.[29] Typical was the Bache Report on steam engines, which was meant to be a practical guide for preventing accidental explosions but which also incorporated the best research available on thermodynamics.

Another major innovation was the formation of national professional associations in science, medicine, and engineering beginning in the 1840s. These organizations encouraged their members to adhere more to peer standards of thinking and behavior (that is, to a scientific research ethos) than to popular understandings such as the Protestant model or the philosophy of useful knowledge.

The growth of the scientific research ethos was rapid in this country. "In the year 1846 nothing like a modern university nor even serious graduate training existed in the United States."[30] Fifteen years later, Yale began to award a Ph.D., and four years after that Cornell opened its doors as a secular school, showing much appreciation for French- and German-style science but none for the Protestant model. The most dramatic moment of all was the 1876 founding of Johns Hopkins University, originally a carbon copy of the German research university. This inspired the 1887 founding of Clark University and the 1891 establishment of the University of Chicago. Equally important, the founding of Johns Hopkins forced every existing liberal arts university, public and private, to choose between a modest role as a liberal arts college or a grand mission as a research university. Most took the latter route.

By the end of the century, says Daniels, the professional goals of most American scientists were to contribute to scientific knowledge (in European terms, that is) and to sustain the scientific community for example, by preparing students for scientific careers.[31] Gone were the "autodictatic amateur" scientists who had sustained the Protestant model.[32] In fact, says Walter Conser, as a result of the professionalization of science in a secular style, most of the Protestant ministry retreated from metaphysical questions about nature's role in verifying faith and turned instead to inner questions of God and conscience.[33]

The scientific research ethos thus had several distinctive values. It was *secular,* that is, uncoupled from religious beliefs regarding purpose or method. It was *rationalist,* employing a positivist attitude and such logical methods as organized skepticism, to reduce knowledge of nature to abstract principles. It was *naturalistic,* requiring that natural phenomena be explained in terms of natural laws or processes. And it recommended *science for the sake of science* in the sense that a career of pure scientific curiosity could be as honorable as any other calling, even if nonscientists felt otherwise. This was also the time when the meaning of the word "science" was narrowed to connote the systematic study of the natural world, thereby displacing such preceding terms as "natural history," "natural philosophy," and "useful arts."

THE CULTURAL FAILURE OF POPULARIZATION

Even though the scientific research ethos gave American scientists great pleasure, making them an esteemed caste of knowledge makers and knowledge organizers and connecting them to the best scientists in the world, it also insulated scientists and their professional values from the rest of American culture. True, the modern scientific research ethos had some good friends among well-educated middle-class and upper-middle-class audiences, but this only emphasized how stratified, how selective, that friendship was. The rest of the American people, which is to say most of the American people, could not or would not embrace the cluster of values joining secularism, rationalism, naturalism, and science for the sake of science. Unlike the Protestant model or useful knowledge, the new model of science was ungrounded in common American values. By the early decades of the twentieth century, a great intellectual gap separated scientists from most of the public.[34]

John Burnham and Marcel LaFollette diagnose this gap as a problem of popularization: with the new scientific ethos unfamiliar to so many Americans, how would it be explained and justified to the public? According to Burnham, the first several generations of scientists to embrace the new ethos made a valiant effort to explain the new values to the American public and even to convert nonscientists to this vision, trying to reach the public directly through learned lectures and high-quality writing. By the 1920s, however, almost all reputable scientists were directing their attention only to their peers, so the mission of popularizing science shifted by default to journalists, advertisers, and science teachers with suspect credentials, none of whom did justice to the core values of the scientific research ethos.[35]

Instead of advocating and explaining the secularist, rationalist, and naturalistic spirit of the new science, the twentieth-century popularizers drew attention to its relatively trivial features. The science journalists, for example, subjected science to mundane journalistic standards. News about science had to be entertaining and, preferably, sensational. It also had to be fast-breaking, as if each day's scientific findings ought to renounce those of the day before. This kind of treatment eviscerated the idea that scientific research was a process of building new knowledge on previous knowledge. It also disembodied scientific facts from the intellectual processes that produced them.

A second common habit of the popularizers was to describe science only in terms of the material end products of the scientific process, that is, gadgets, drugs, or weapons. This, of course, treated the scientific research ethos as a mere extension of the philosophy of useful knowledge, as if the new style of science had no distinctive core values of its own. At a time when the public ought to have been considering those core values and weighing them against the values of the Protestant model and useful knowledge, those values became all but invisible relative to the parade of gadgets that supposedly represented science.

A third habit of the popularizers, including the science teachers, was to erase the more arduous features of learning—namely, mathematics and mastery of empirical detail—from popular images of science. To science journalists, those features were insufficiently entertaining. To science teachers, the discipline required to master math and empirical detail violated a sacred tenet of American educational philosophy: each student possessed a certain innate individual potential. Thus, the purpose of formal education was to celebrate and enhance each student's individual gifts. By that standard, discipline was regimentation, and regimentation was un-American.

In short, the process of popularizing the new style of science shattered the public understanding of that science into bits of trivia, reports of gadgets, and other piddling matters far removed from the virtues of secularism, rationalism, and naturalism, let alone science for the sake of science. While the scientific community became increasingly sophisticated intellectually, the rest of America received the worst possible message about the place of science in our lives. "Science in the realm of the popularizers," writes Burnham, "changed from a coherent view of nature, including humans, into choppy, unconnected 'facts.'" "The cultural symbolism of science disintegrated—the view that science stood for something."[36]

Surely it was difficult enough to explain the scientific research ethos to the American public, given that the model was novel and that it was a European import. Surely the ethos needed all the help it could get if it was going to somehow fit into a larger framework of common American cultural values. Instead, the scientific research ethos was subjected to a dreadful process of popularization that subverted the public's understanding of its unique worth.

Then again, the mischief of the popularizers was not the only force that undermined appreciation of the new research ethos. That ethos itself, in its purest ivory-tower way of thinking, discouraged its practitioners from justifying their work to the general population on the grounds that a good relation with nonscientists might represent an end run around scientific standards. One could be either a good scientist or a cheap popularizer but not both. That was the choice forced on the acolytes of the scientific research ethos. And that helps explain why the the process of popularization was such a failure. It was subcontracted by default from those who could best articulate the new ethos to those who were least prepared to advocate its intellectual spirit.

Another serious problem was the chronic condition of American science education. Although this calling has had highlights, cycles of reform, and moments of optimism in its history, each generation of public school science teachers faces the same timeless obstacles. One is that the content of the science curriculum answers more to the parochial standards of local and state school boards than to the judgments of the scientific community. Another is that science is expensive to teach, both in time and equipment. Superficial science education, based on textbooks and lectures, is far more affordable than substantive learning anchored in the many activities of discovery. Finally, science education tolerates mediocrity much more than science does, if only because a public school has to pass most of its students. If science education is the gateway to an understanding of the scientific research ethos, then that ethos is poorly served.

A stark example is Judith Grabiner and Peter Miller's account of the place of evolution in science education. After the Scopes trial of 1925, when creationism was humiliated and discredited, the American scientific community invested great confidence in the study of evolution, as if the results of the Scopes trial were general and eternal. Meanwhile, evolution was largely purged from public school science because state and local school boards feared the kinds of controversy that had descended on Dayton, Tennessee, site of the Scopes trial, and because science textbook publishers mirrored the apprehensions of the school boards. This purging had nothing to do with the scientific merits of either evolution or creationism. It was a democratic process that guaranteed that science did not intrude too much into science education. And so, according to Grabiner and Miller, "the evolutionists of the 1920s believed they had won a great victory in the Scopes trial. But as far as teaching biology in the high schools was concerned, they had not won; they had lost. Not only did they lose, but they did not even know they had lost."[37]

One final problem was that the audience for science was greatly fragmented. The Protestant model might touch anyone who saw virtue or revelation in Protestant terms, and the philosophy of useful knowledge could please all those who embraced prosperity or democracy or independence or any combination thereof. But the scientific research ethos had a relatively small natural constituency—namely, the part of the population that wanted the systematic study of nature to be secular, rationalist, and naturalistic. One did not have to be a professional scientist to feel this way, but one surely had to be intellectually different from most of one's American neighbors. So there developed one form of written and spoken communication for scientists addressing scientists; another form pitched to nonscientists friendly to the research ethos; a third form for the general public, embodying all the journalistic vices just mentioned; and a fourth form for children, that is, the stylistics of science education.[38]

That last point should remind us that we now have an enduring situation in which three very different visions of science circulate in American life. Of these, the philosophy of useful knowledge is undoubtedly the best integrated into the common themes of American culture since the fruits this model is expected to yield—progress, democracy, and independence—are as desirable today as they were two hundred years ago. The Protestant model has receded far from its original influence, both because the larger culture has become much more secular and because most Protestants want to dedicate their faith to matters much more pressing than arguing with modern science about how to study nature. Nevertheless, the Protestant model also has a certain staying power of its own, as manifested in the popularity of "scientific creationism," which is an elaborate update of that model.

Then there is the European Enlightenment scientific research ethos. Although it has captured the minds of most American scientists, this ethos has hardly purged the two former systems of belief from American life. Then and now, it is normal to want science to be virtuous and useful. The research ethos is virtuous, but only in its own terms, and useful, but only sometimes. The other two models are much better grounded in obvious virtue and tangible usefulness than the newer vision of science. The research ethos exists within American culture, which is big and roomy, but it is connected only loosely, if at all, to the moral landmarks of that culture.

This brief history of science in American culture also means, ironically, that conditions for the conjuring of science come not from the two earlier visions of science and nature but from the rise of *modern* science. Even if the substance of the scientific research ethos was not much understood by most of the American public, that ethos nevertheless earned their respect, which I have called "science in an Old Testament style." The fault, I think, lies in the failure of the process of popularization rather than in the science itself, but regardless of where we assign the blame, we have to see that the modern vision of science endures an affliction that the previous two models did not. Its intellectual substance is alien to large parts of the general population, whereas the common symbols of this ethos are borrowed from a different vision of nature and science, namely, the philosophy of useful knowledge. Given that the conjuring of science is a kind of troublemaking that takes place in the gap between the substance of science and its symbols, the scientific research ethos is far more vulnerable to this mischief than its two predecessors, the Protestant model and useful knowledge.

CHAPTER THREE

■ ■ ■

Democratic Culture and the Moral Autonomy of Science

The cultural failure of popularization was far from obvious in its early days late in the nineteenth century and well into the first half of the twentieth. In fact, there were ways to get around that failure. Joseph Henry and some other scientists in the U.S. government justified their work, which they conducted in the spirit of the new scientific research ethos, by referring to the philosophy of useful knowledge; they promised tangible results while discreetly pursuing their own private plans of theoretical research. After all, they reasoned, the science of the new ethos was good science, but it could not be justified as such to voters, taxpayers, and elected officials.[1]

This attitude was fine when hard results were plentiful and obvious but not so fine when the fruits of the new science were more abstract: thoughts about relativity, uncertainty, and the Hubble Constant or geology's hypothetical reconstructions of life on earth long ago. This attitude was also not so fine when scientists were candid about *scientia gratia scientiae* (science for the sake of science). Then the philosophy of useful knowledge broke down as a cover for the scientific research ethos, thereby exposing again the problem of fitting the new ethos into the main currents of American culture.

The intellectual friends of the scientific research ethos, most of whom were not scientists per se, gave much thought to that question about science and American culture. In doing so, they affirmed that love is blind, for they saw only the virtues of the scientific ethos that had captured their hearts, and they celebrated its virtues by generating a pair of naively optimistic theories about science and American culture. These two theories, which I call the "moral autonomy theory" (meaning that the morality of science stands apart from the morality of the larger culture) and the "enhancement theory" (meaning that science and democracy automatically enhance each other), both overlooked the possibility that the scientific research ethos might be incompatible with American democratic culture. The unintended effect of both was to aggravate the conditions that permitted the conjuring of science by underestimating the cultural failure of popularization.

THE MORAL AUTONOMY OF SCIENCE

One kind of logic, more European than American, held that science deserved special exemptions from democratic processes—that is, "self-rule for science, support without strings, the time and money to do research without having to account to laymen for its direction or consequences."[2] That had been one of the foundation stones of the Continental scientific culture, which American scientists greatly envied.

This dream that science might call its own shots and be autonomous even from its benefactors was as old as the earliest American efforts to establish European scientific practices on this side of the Atlantic in the 1840s. But the idea had scant plausibility in the land of the Protestant model and useful knowledge until the 1940s, when two lines of justification arose, one of them intellectual, the other a fact of government policy.

The first line of justification developed as a reaction to German fascism's startling claims about science as a handmaiden to ideology. "Racial hygiene," "German physics," and other strange projects irritated American intellectuals and offended them greatly. Racial hygiene, the project of Josef Mengele and his associates, pretended to reveal sharp anatomical differences separating ethnic Germans from other peoples, especially Jews. "German physics" was little more than a categorical denunciation of "Jewish physics," meaning Einsteinian relativity. American intellectuals knew instinctively that these exercises in Nazi science were greatly flawed both scientifically and morally.[3] But how should intellectuals refute the Nazi claims that science substantiated Nazi thought?

One strategy might have been to argue these issues in empirical detail, disproving specific hypotheses or discrediting particular experiments. This, of course, required a certain level of scientific expertise. But the most agitated critics of Nazi science were intellectual friends of science who lacked the skills and credentials to challenge Nazi sciencc. Many an American scientist was apolitical, for the more extreme interpretation of science-for-the-sake-of-science demanded that scientists be detached from political issues. Another complication might have been that the racial hygienists in Germany had strong affinities to British and American eugenicists of recent decades, in which case the particulars of German fascist thought would not be easily disentangled from science in the democratic societies.

A second strategy grew out of a sense of political morality. Since Nazi science was obviously an uncritical extension of Nazi political thought, the basic problem could be described as the general relationship of science and government as posited by the Nazi state. If it could be shown that democratic values were friendlier to science than were the values of the German fascists, implying that democratic culture nurtured better science than fascist culture, then the Nazi claims about "racial hygiene" and "German physics" would be broken. This enterprise required fairly broad definitions of scientific and political values.

The most influential argument to emerge from this sense of political morality was that of sociologist Robert Merton, who described a four-part "normative structure of science" in a pair of essays on "science and democratic social structure" published in 1938 and 1942.[4] Merton argued that the institution of science was regulated by four internal values: universalism, communal ownership of knowledge, disinterestedness, and organized skepticism. It was especially obvious that universalism was alien to Nazi thought. As defined by Merton, universalism meant that science should be open to all kinds of people— Jews for instance—without regard to race, religion, or ethnicity. But his discussions also implied that the other three values digressed from fascism. Disinterestedness put a wall between science and ideology. Communal ownership of scientific knowledge contrasted with state control of such knowledge. Organized skepticism opposed the blind obedience expected within German fascism.

Along with these four normative values came strong social pressures to conform to them, with the result, in Merton's theory, that the actual behavior of most scientists was faithful to these values. This way, nonscientists would easily see that science as an institution had considerable intrinsic moral worth and that its normative structure was absolutely incompatible with that of a totalitarian government.[5] By isolating and celebrating the intrinsic merits of science, this formulation emphasized that the institution of science was morally autonomous.

Merton depicted science as a very virtuous institution, but he also portrayed it as a moral system unlike other moral systems since no other moral system comprised this same combination of normative values.

What, then, was the proper relation of science to society? According to Merton's reasoning, the proper course was for a society to nurture the work of scientists without interfering in their internal relations because the scientific community, by virtue of its own special normative structure, had sufficient moral authority to police its own affairs. Other communities in a society—that is, nonscientists—lacked the authority to pass judgment on science because they were uninvolved in scientific values. Most important, Merton implied that a democracy would support science without interfering in its work but a fascist state could not resist using science as an extension of its political ideology. Taken to an extreme, this view suggested that it was undemocratic for any government, even a democracy, to hold scientists accountable to external values.

I do not mean to imply that all the merits and faults of this theory are solely attributable to Robert Merton, like Athena and her wisdom springing fully grown from the brow of Zeus. These thoughts circulated among alarmed leftists during the rise of German fascism. Nevertheless, Merton put that sentiment into words more effectively than others. His moral autonomy theory has since become the foundation of mainstream sociology of science.[6] An example is *The Scientist's Role in Society,* wherein Joseph Ben-David offered a historical and comparative account of the rise of science in Western civilization. According to Ben-David, two conditions were necessary for modern science: society made the role of the scientist a legitimate role by deeming it a respectable profession, and society's support for science was decentralized, so that the scientist had all the academic freedom he or she needed.[7] On this basis, Ben-David praised those situations that gave scientists the most prestige with the least direct accountability, and he scorned those that did the opposite. His work was a detailed amplification of the Merton thesis, including the idea that nonscientists need only respect science, not understand it.

A much more influential manifestation of the autonomy theory was American postwar science policy as recommended by Vannevar Bush, science adviser to Presidents Franklin Roosevelt and Harry Truman. In the 1945 report *Science, the Endless Frontier,* Bush argued that the federal government ought to assume primary responsibility for supporting scientific research. At that time this argument signaled an extraordinary expansion of government support for science, and the foremost result was the eventual creation of the National Science Foundation. Bush also recommended minimal interference from the government and maximum freedom for the scientist.[8] As if echoing Merton, Bush wrote:

> Scientific progress on a broad front results from the free play of free intellects, working on subjects of their own choice, in the manner dictated by their curiosity for exploration of the unknown. . . . Support of basic research in the public and private colleges, universities, and research institutes must leave the internal control of policy, personnel, and the method and scope of the research to the institutions themselves. This is of utmost importance.[9]

Compared with other government programs, Bush's plan was an unprecedented suspension of the recipients' accountability to taxpayers and voters. President Truman complained that an autonomous National Science Foundation would be "divorced from control by the people to an extent that it implies a distinct lack of faith in democratic processes."[10] Regardless, Bush's recommendations were adopted, and for forty years or so they set the tone for U.S. government support of basic scientific research. In the Manhattan Project the autonomy model was developed, in the Atomic Energy Act of 1946 it was enshrined, and in the arrangement known as the "administrative contract," it was institutionalized. Basic science received special conditions of freedom and flexibility that insulated it from meddling bureaucrats, political mischief, and external influence in general.[11] Thus did U.S. government science policy converge with Robert Merton's theory.

THE DEMISE OF THE MORAL AUTONOMY OF SCIENCE

The moral autonomy model cannot account for the possibility that a democracy might do to a scientific question what it does to other questions: subject it to a democratic decision-making process. A general vote on a scientific question is preposterous, according to the autonomy model. Historians George Daniels and Nathan Reingold have cautioned that the autonomy model is in the long run unrealistic and likely to lead to trouble. It is an "undemocratic suspension of the rules," says Daniels, who feels that if science depends on financial support from the public via the government, then "it must seek some means of contact with the values of the enveloping society."[12] Reingold warns that "it is naive to hope for and to expect immunity from the ebb and flow of history."[13] Like it or not, a democracy sometimes takes an active interest in scientific questions, even if the results are messy.

The predictions of Daniels and Reingold have recently come to life in a most unpleasant form. Throughout the 1960s and 1970s, Senator William Proxmire's "Golden Fleece Award" was the usual style of congressional criticism of government-funded scientific research. Proxmire would select an esoteric-sounding grant and then ridicule it for being highfalutin or for supposedly investigating the obvious. This was the Common Sense philosophy at its bluntest: if a nonscientist does not appreciate the research, then it must be worthless, in which case the scientist must be fleecing the taxpayer. In retrospect, however, Proxmire's criticism was relatively mild, for he only claimed that a scientist's research was foolish, not criminal, and he highlighted individual grants without implying that science in general was troubled.

During the 1980s, however, congressional respect for the moral autonomy of science evaporated as Representative John Dingell began a series of very aggressive investigations of scientists and research institutions that made Proxmire's approach seem mild by comparison.[14] For instance, the case of Tereza Imanishi-Kari and David Baltimore versus Margot O'Toole began as a legitimate difference of opinion about interpreting data from an experiment that sought to affect antibodies by introducing a foreign gene. But with the benefit of Dingell's investigation, this disagreement escalated into a full-blown accusation that Imanishi-Kari and Baltimore had committed serious, blatant fraud. Before this conflict was over, Nobel laureate Baltimore was very thoroughly and very publicly humiliated.

Similarly, there is reason to believe that when the National Institutes of Health (NIH) investigated Robert Gallo for claiming undue credit for discovering the HIV virus, the investigators were pressured by Dingell and his staff to judge Gallo more harshly than they would have otherwise, as they had indeed done in the Baltimore case.[15] When it seemed to Dingell that NIH director Bernadine Healy was obstructing the Gallo investigation, he resurrected unrelated charges that Healy had mishandled a previous investigation. Furthermore, Dingell's investigation of overhead charges at Stanford University contributed to Donald Kennedy's decision to resign as president of that school, and it also raised fears of a widespread overhead scandal, as numerous research universities suddenly recalculated their indirect costs.

In truth, Dingell was not concerned exclusively with scientists. He had been equally harsh with bank regulators, the insurance industry, cable TV companies, and Pentagon procurement officers. Nevertheless, the consequences for the moral credibility of science were especially awful. Never before in American history were so many scientists subjected to withering public accusations of fraud, corruption, conflict of interest, and other kinds of conduct bordering on the criminal. The cumulative effect was a generalized suspicion that science as an institution could not deal with its members' misconduct.[16] Dingell's investigators presumed that scientists in general were "stubborn and corrupt individuals" who habitually lied and concealed evidence; "from the [investigations] subcommittee there emanated a deep animus against this country's scientific establishment."[17] As a result, Dingell's staff felt that David Baltimore had to be publicly humiliated as a lesson to all scientists.

Representative Dingell's accusations, which were sometimes valid, sometimes not, strike at the heart of the theory that science is morally autonomous. "Scientists are not very persuasive when they argue that politicians have no business in scientific affairs."[18] Investigations like Dingell's have the power to "establish a climate that is anathema to high-quality scientific research" and "diminish the morale, attractiveness and authority" of science when uncertainties, hunches, and judgments are depicted as criminal behavior.[19] Suzanne Garment says that our political culture has an insatiable hunger for scandal.[20] If the institution of science is like a newly discovered continent, until recently off limits to external accusations of scandal, then science offers enormous new opportunities to aggressive accusers, predatory investigators, and zealous prosecutors.

Distrust of scientists also comes from outside the government, and Randy Shilts's political history of the AIDS epidemic illustrates this kind of hostility. In Shilts's story, frontline epidemiologists at the Centers for Disease Control are heroes, and so are clinicians who treat people with AIDS. But research scientists at the National Institutes of Health are generally indifferent to the AIDS epidemic and condescending to those who care about it. In September 1981, says Shilts, the NIH scientists "didn't care [about AIDS], because there was little glory, fame, and funding in this field."[21] The author describes the research ethos at NIH this way: "Pure science. That means nobody can tell them what to do. The scientists follow their own interests, and, it is hoped, they will stumble across discoveries that will benefit mankind."[22] After suggesting repeatedly that ivory-tower intellectuals at NIH had subverted the fight against AIDS by retarding the pace of research for the pettiest of reasons, Shilts adds sardonically that they justified their unconscionable behavior by describing it as "scientifically responsible" and "responsible science."[23]

Another blow against the autonomy of science, particularly federally funded science, came from the painful discovery of economic limitations in the 1990s. President George Bush's science adviser, D. Allan Bromley, ended his term by warning that the age of expansion in academic research had ended and that many research programs needed to be cut.[24] The same kind of sentiment was also evident in Congress, where few members felt that scientific autonomy took precedence over economic difficulties.[25] The demise of the superconducting supercollider, which offered hard promises about abstract knowledge but only vague allusions to useful knowledge, was a clear sign that science for the sake of science was in for bad weather.[26]

With hindsight, we can see that the autonomy theory, whether described in the theories of Robert Merton or executed in the policies of the U.S. government, was unrealistic about the articulation of scientific values with American democratic culture. It underestimated the latter, especially the democratic ethos that funding from the public requires accountability to the public. Admittedly, the theory worked to the advantage of scientists for many decades, but now that this era is coming to a close, we can see that a certain grand folly was concealed within the moral autonomy theory: as long as the public trusted science, it did not matter to scientists whether the public understood science. This way, the moral autonomy of science helped create science in an Old Testament style, that is, respect without comprehension. When it was unimportant whether the public understood the intellectual substance of science, nonscientists came to know science only in terms of mysterious symbols that stood for science.

SCIENCE'S ENHANCEMENT OF DEMOCRACY

A second way of connecting science with American democratic culture was the idea that scientific thinking automatically enhanced that culture, as if science were the spiritual core of democracy. This was the logical opposite of the moral autonomy theory, but it, too, had adverse consequences for public understanding of the new scientific research ethos because it surrounded that ethos with näiveté, fuzzy thinking, and unrealistic expectations.

This theory, that science enhanced democracy, consisted largely of a style of thinking: when American intellectuals were optimistic about the quality of life, they included science within that spirit of optimism. The social and political reformers of the early twentieth century believed that American government worked well. Those who enjoyed the middle-class prosperity of the industrial age were optimistic that a better life was at hand. Many American intellectuals, especially those associated with John Dewey, connected reform and prosperity with science by arguing that the philosophical core of democracy and prosperity was a cluster of liberal and humanistic values, with scientific thinking at the center of these values.

There were three ways to include science in this sense of optimism. One was to attribute prosperity to science, which was yet another resurrection of the philosophy of useful knowledge, equating science with technology.[27] The other two approaches depended on the European Enlightenment model of science, for they suggested that rationalist thought, borrowed directly from science, guided success and happiness. One of these postulated that good government was based on scientific principles and methods, especially experimental methods. The other was a more general belief that scientific thinking would enhance the intangible qualities of American life by, among other results, emancipating citizens' minds.[28]

The American style of government is, to say the least, experimental, for it has a great propensity to tinker, to change, to reform. Abraham Lincoln, for instance, made good use of the metaphor of government-as-an-experiment.[29] Don Price and other scholars have interpreted the American style of government as an exercise in scientific methods of experimentation by saying that "American democracy is the political version of the scientific method."[30]

In a very sophisticated variation of this thesis, Yaron Ezrahi argues that the cultural value of the visual symbols of liberal democracy is based on the empiricist theories of sense perception postulated by Isaac Newton and John Locke in early-eighteenth-century England. Popular faith in science was enhanced when it was visually demystified: that is, when the public could directly observe experiments and demonstrations. People could understand what they could see, and they could support what they could understand. Subsequently, says Ezrahi, this insight was extended to liberal-democratic government: the visual imagery of government should appeal not only to ruling elites but also to the larger population, which was quite a novel insight in the time of Newton and Locke.[31]

And yet theories like Price's, which trace an experimental style of government directly to an experimental style of science, are ultimately tracing the former to the methodology of the nineteenth-century German research universities. It seems to me that this theory gives too much credit to science and not enough to the unorganized uniqueness of American history. The instances in which American government has been explicitly modeled on science are rare; those in which governmental method unintentionally resembles scientific method are only coincidences. Ideally, it is good for government to benefit from scientific knowledge and methods, but ultimately government has a dynamic life of its own in which the goodness of government derives from much else besides science.

According to the more general approach, science enhances democracy by providing mental models for everyday life.[32] John Dewey felt that the way for individuals and groups to benefit from experience was to embrace scientific methods. Not to do so, he felt, was to surrender to "the entrenched and stubborn institutions of the past."[33] "The fundamental problem," he wrote, was "unwillingness to adopt the scientific attitude."[34] Dewey insisted that progress required scientific thinking: "Ultimately and philosophically, science is the organ of general social progress."[35] Also, "great as have been the social changes of the last century, they are not to be compared with those which will emerge when our faith in scientific method is more manifest in social works."[36] In a similar spirit, Karl Popper reacted to the rise of Nazism and Stalinism by drawing a sharp contrast between democracy and totalitarianism according to which the former could be expected to use experimental methods borrowed from science, whereas the latter typically distorted science.[37]

Theories that linked science to democratic culture were often vague about the form of progress that would result from the link. When progress was understood simply in terms of material prosperity, the enhancement theory was badly shaken by the Great Depression, for it then seemed that science was powerless to reestablish the prosperity of earlier times. By the 1950s, however, there was enormous satisfaction that democracy and science had together solved the classic socioeconomic questions that had tormented the industrial societies. The satisfaction was so great that Daniel Bell could announce "the end of ideology."[38]

THE CREDIBILITY OF THE ENHANCEMENT THEORY

But where does all this scientific thinking come from? This is a serious problem with the enhancement theory. If the source is unspecified, then science is a disembodied *Geist* (spirit), present everywhere but coming from nowhere. But if science really infuses American democratic culture and enhances it, then scientific thinking has to be located in the citizenry. It must be that the adult members of this democracy have some scientific knowledge from which they form the scientific judgments that supposedly enhance democracy. And if they have sufficient scientific knowledge to think scientifically about government and the quality of life, then presumably they are able to apply that knowledge to issues of science policy as well, not necessarily as experts, but at least as informed participants in the democratic process. "Although only a few may originate a policy, we are all able to judge it"—thus said Pericles, and thus was he quoted by Karl Popper to illustrate the place of science in democratic culture.[39]

If all this is so, then the enhancement theory is hopelessly unrealistic. A series of polls by Jon Miller reveals that "a substantial majority of the electorate are ill-prepared to make . . . judgments" in referendums and controversies about nuclear power, Laetrile, recombinant DNA, and fluoridation.[40] Miller reports that the level of scientific literacy in the United States is less than 10 percent of the adult population, which is "dreadfully low," and reflects "widespread confusion about scientific terms."[41] Large numbers of adult Americans "don't know enough to understand basic discussions about scientific research" and "cannot distinguish between science and pseudoscience."[42]

Science journalism often aggravates the problem of scientific illiteracy. Dorothy Nelkin finds that science journalism typically substitutes shallow imagery for substantive content and that it frames science stories with dramatic hyperbole.[43] Although science journalism has greatly increased the *quantity* of scientific information that reaches nonscientists, this is very different, Nelkin notes, from improving the *quality* of scientific understanding.[44] Magic, mystery, hope, and fear are the main themes of most science journalism.[45] Similarly, John Burnham reports that the history of science journalism is equivalent to a long-term process of trivializing and fragmenting the public understanding of science.[46] And Allan Mazur's study of several scientific disputes shows that, ironically, an increase in the quantity of media attention leads to an increase in hostility toward the science or technology in question, probably because the media unintentionally inflame fears of technological catastrophe.[47]

The implications of these findings are not subtle. Scientific thinking can hardly enhance democratic culture when barely anyone can think scientifically. As Michael Shortland puts it, "If the general public is to have a voice in scientific decision-making, then it had better know something about the science whose future it is helping to decide."[48] He is quite right, but the truth about scientific literacy indicates that well-informed science policy is beyond the scope of the democratic decision-making process.[49]

Science education, which is a necessary precondition for scientific literacy, brings equally bad news.[50] Standardized tests that compare American children with foreigners of the same age reveal two patterns: (1) the abilities of American children in science and math are distinctly inferior to those of many Asians and Europeans, and, (2) these abilities decline for American children (relative to the children of other nations) as they move through the school system. According to a study reported in 1988, American fourteen-year-olds placed fourteenth out of seventeen nations in science achievement.[51] A 1989 report showed American thirteen-year-olds performing "dead last" in math among twenty nations.[52] In a comparison of Chinese and American first-graders, the former were faster at solving mathematical problems and used more sophisticated methods, and in a four-nation comparison American fifth-graders had math scores lower than those for China, Taiwan, and Japan.[53] Generally, American children are "significantly below the mean" in these multinational tests.[54] When several grades are tested at the same time, then the American children's relative achievement in science and math grows worse from grade to grade.[55]

The consequence is that most Americans are not ready for science in college or for technology at work. Only about 7 percent of American seventeen-year-olds are "adequately prepared for college-level science courses," and more than half of them "have so little scientific understanding that they cannot hold down jobs that require technical skills . . . or make informed decisions as citizens."[56] In short, "a reexamination of how science is represented and studied is required."[57]

By contrast, science education in Japan, Germany, China, and the former Soviet Union is distinctly more successful because those nations are committed to high standards and priorities for science education in planning and policy. For the United States, there is "no comparable commitment," and in fact American leadership in this area is "sporadic."[58]

Students' feelings about science, as measured in periodic surveys, reflect the unhappy state of science education. Margaret Mead and Rhoda Metraux reported in 1957 that high school students had a positive opinion of science in general, but "when the question becomes one of . . . science as a career choice . . . the image is overwhelmingly negative."[59] Students saw science as tedious and scientists as saintly but dull. Girls feared that male scientists made bad husbands. Four years later, David Beardslee and Donald O'Dowd found much the same attitudes among college students, with scientists believed to be "unsociable, introverted, and possessing few, if any, friends."[60] A scientist was thought to have an "unhappy home life, and a wife who is not pretty."[61] In 1975 Michael Shallis and Philip Hills described a more varied spectrum of young people's perceptions of scientists, that is, friendly, neutral, and hostile images, but even the neutral image held that scientists were reserved, remote, and unable to explain their work to the public.[62]

The theory that science enhances democratic culture is very attractive. Surely democracy is a good way to make decisions; surely science is a good way to know nature. If goodness is cut from whole cloth, then, of course, one enhances the other. And if citizens know enough about science to think more or less like scientists, then no one could get away with conjuring science by switching the symbols of science for its substance.

The evidence, however, hardly supports the theory. Considering how scant, feeble, and fragmented scientific understanding is in this society, no one can plausibly argue that most Americans think scientifically about government and the quality of life, let alone use that kind of thinking to guide their behavior. The miserable condition of scientific literacy, science education, and science journalism demonstrates that scientific thinking has very little democratic grounding in the general population. Timothy Ferris asks, "Is it really plausible to assert that science permeates an American society in which only one in five high-school graduates has taken a physics course, only one in four has heard that the universe is expanding, 21 percent think the sun orbits the earth, and nearly half the public believes that 'God created man pretty much in his present form at one time within the last 10,000 years'?"[63]

A fundamental premise of political culture holds that an informed electorate is a necessary condition for democracy. But the premise is moot if scientific authority is invoked to help resolve an issue but the scientific literacy of the electorate is too shallow to comprehend that authority. The core of the enhancement theory, that the good things about our government and our quality of life can be attributed to citizens reasoning like scientists, is not credible.

DEMOCRATIC SCIENCE

But citizens will reason *about* science anyway, even if they do not reason like scientists. Given that they will participate in decisions about science, thus contradicting the moral autonomy theory, and given the realities of science education, scientific literacy, and science journalism, which together subvert the theory that science enhances democracy, then how should we describe the place of science in American democratic culture?

Edward Larson describes "public science" as the common ground where nonscientists' understandings of science meet those of scientists—that is, in publicly supported science education and related activities that are inevitably affected by public opinion.[64] He emphasizes that the opinions of scientists have limited impact, even in science education, because other points of view are also influential, especially those of legislatures, judges, and school boards, which often have nonscientific criteria for making decisions about science and science education.[65] A scientific issue, says Larson, cannot be resolved through legal measures if it cannot be settled in public opinion.[66] In fact, questions of science policy, like those of science education, are also questions of the democratic process because nonscientists are inevitably involved in them.

To expand Larson's insights a little, I propose the idea of "democratic science": that is, a matrix of cultural conditions (including values, meanings, symbols, judgments, and the opinions of nonscientists) in which both the style and the content of science are shaped by direct and indirect democratic processes, including elections, referenda, legislation, litigation, consensus, and compromise. Nonscientists' understandings of science intersect with the expertise of credentialed scientists, and scientific thought is subject to extrascientific considerations. The subject matter is science, but the framework is American democratic culture. As defined, democratic science includes the following considerations:

School board decisions about the content of science education

Referendums on fluoridation and other scientific policies

The role of scientists as expert witnesses

Campaigns to persuade the government to expedite approval of a particular drug, such as DMSO, Laetrile, or AZT, or to fund a particular program of research and development, as in the case of cold fusion

The deployment of scientists' testimony when legislatures and courts consider waste disposal, electromagnetic fields, and other modern technologies

And so if the procedures of democratic science are how decisions about science are made, and how thought about science is nurtured in this democratic culture, then the question of how people understand science is hardly a simple matter of scientists handing knowledge to students and adults. Instead, it is a messy problem in which various forms of the Protestant model, useful knowledge, and the scientific research ethos compete for attention and credibility. (Useful knowledge, in one form or another, usually wins.) Scientists embracing the research ethos have the right to advocate their kind of science, but their efforts are handicapped when they embrace discredited ideas such as the enhancement theory and the moral autonomy theory.

This discussion of democratic science raises other questions: Are these problems unique to *American* democratic culture? Or are they common to democracies in general? Do other democratic cultures have other ways of fitting science into people's lives? This is a good anthropological question of cross-cultural comparison. A group of political scientists, not waiting for anthropologists to get to it, have posed this question and have found some provocative answers.

Denmark produces a series of "consensus conferences" in which a small group of nonscientists studies a current scientific issue carefully over many months and then offers an informed opinion. The government's Board of Technology names the topic and then assembles a panel that represents the nation's population, more or less, but excludes experts who have a direct interest in the topic. The Board of Technology gets the group started with a background paper and other materials, but then the group seeks its own information, including expert testimony. The final result is a statement by nonexperts about the issue at hand. As an opinion, it is not legally binding, but as a consensus position by nonscientists on a current scientific issue, it is extremely informative to policy makers and interest groups.[67]

The Netherlands offers a network of fifty "science shops" in which university scientists make their expertise available to nonprofit organizations. The organizations approach the shops with such concerns as pollution or worker safety. When the shops provide useful knowledge about a given problem, this process teaches the scientists much about the needs and the curiosity of the public and assures the nonprofit organizations that science can enhance people's lives.[68]

Sweden has pioneered a "Scandinavian Approach" to technological change in the workplace: all parties, including workers, with a stake in a given change participate in all phases of the decision-making process, including the design phase at the beginning of the process. Some participants have more technological expertise than others, but having less is not grounds for exclusion from decisionmaking. On the contrary, change goes better when it takes into account all levels of expertise. Furthermore, the Scandinavian Approach reveals that those with more modest backgrounds can quickly increase their expertise when necessary.[69]

Langdon Winner gives an illustration of how this approach can make a difference. When a business buys enhanced computer software, graphics, for example, the company may buy U.S.-made packages that can do almost everything. But these are "deskilling" products that make employees insignificant relative to the software. The humans have to fit the software, so to speak. If, however, the business takes employees' skills into account by including employees in the decision-making process from the beginning, then the software has to fit the humans. The business gets better computer graphics, the employees improve their expertise in computer graphics, the technological change in question serves the needs of all parties, and all parties are then committed to making that change work well. "Ordinary people," says Winner, "regardless of background or prior expertise, are capable of taking a turn making decisions of this kind."[70]

The Danish consensus conferences, the Dutch science shops, and the Scandinavian Approach have inspired similar projects in other industrial democracies.[71] Together they indicate that science can find a constructive role in democratic culture using democratic processes. The explicit justification is the philosophy of useful knowledge, but the conferences, the science shops, and the Scandinavian Approach also make good use of the knowledge that comes from the scientific research ethos.

Can these approaches be taken in the United States? If not, can our culture find other democratic methods for fitting science into people's lives? Langdon Winner has long argued that, instead of reacting after the fact to the social and political consequences of technological change, we can anticipate its consequences, and we can then make choices about how it will affect our lives before the consequences are forced on us.[72] Americans are like Scandinavians, he suggests. We can become more sophisticated about science and technology when we have to, but it usually takes a crisis—hazardous waste, ugly pollution, or threats to property values—before this happens. "When faced with threats to their well-being, [American] citizens can quickly become expert in handling technical details and clever in political maneuvering."[73]

Could this kind of quickly acquired expertise be the enhancement theory, in the flesh? True, it shows a *potential* to realize that theory, but there is a catch or two. It is one thing for most citizens to be scientifically literate on a regular basis—the enhancement theory—and yet another for a small group of neighbors reacting to a sudden threat to quickly master a special scientific problem. In addition, American society's preferred method for resolving conflict is litigation. The principal process for making public decisions about science and technology, or about anything else, tends to be highly contentious and adversarial. Litigation also celebrates expert scientific knowledge, thereby devaluing the existential pains of the rest of us whose lives are touched by science and technology. Compromise, although common enough in the litigation process, is far different from consensus. As a result, too often too many citizens are understandably unhappy with public decisions about science and technology. After all, we are only "muddling through" these issues without resolving them in terms of right or wrong.[74] This is democratic science.

How, then, does science makes sense to Americans so that we make it a part of our lives, but only very selectively? To pursue this question, we need to convert the historical problem of science in American life into an anthropological problem by constructing an anthropology of science.

PART TWO

■ ■ ■

An Anthropology of Science

CHAPTER FOUR

■ ■ ■

Scientific Symbols and Cultural Meanings

Most of us who pick apart the meaning of science—writer, readers, reviewers, and those who can artfully fake some knowledge of this book without having read it—are postmodernists. We feel that the intrinsic merits and extrinsic benefits of science are less obvious than our teachers and parents once thought. We know that scientific knowledge does not automatically enhance our lives and that the scientific method is the wrong model for humanistic questions. Likewise, we realize that science may well be distorted as individuals borrow jagged pieces of it to brace one belief or another by appealing to the plenary authority of science.

Still, even if many of us see science through the dark glass of postmodernism, we do so in different forms and to different degrees. Unfortunately, the rhetoric of postmodernism is sometimes fuzzy, obscuring differences of form or degree and making it easy for the reader to infer much when the writer implies little. Terms like "problematize," "deconstruct," "hegemonic discourse," and my own morbid favorite, "phallocentric," can evoke most everything without necessarily signifying anything. Here we have the most cryptic of passwords and codewords, which, like the muffled lyrics of "Louie, Louie," let us think what we will without asking writers or readers to say what they mean.

But as I convert my historical observations on science into an anthropological problem, I should clarify my own preferences, lest readers rush to the conclusion that my postmodernist preferences are the same as theirs. Mine are those of a school of cultural anthropology known as "interpretive anthropology," so called because its program is to interpret the symbols found in human culture in light of the meanings behind them and to interpret the meanings that steer our lives in terms of the symbols that make them manifest.

MEANINGS AND SYMBOLS

Together we make sense of our lives by creating and sharing moralities, philosophies, ideologies, beliefs, and values, which is to say that human culture has existential substance. "Meanings" is the cultural anthropologist's term for this substance. These meanings, however, are intangible. To understand them, to act on them, and to communicate them to others, we need tangible and visual symbols: stories, rituals, images, emblems, slogans, virtues, and role models.

A given culture is a particular matrix of meanings and symbols by which a group of people makes sense of the world around them. In the words of Clifford Geertz, symbols are "abstractions from experience fixed in perceptible forms."[1] Their function, writes James Peacock, "is to express a configuration of consciousness."[2]

Ideally, the relation between meaning and symbol is simple, clear, and stable. Typically, however, it is problematic. Symbols are "polysemic": they are capable of conveying multiple different meanings so that the same image means different things to different people. Or a relationship of meaning and symbol might change over time so that a given symbol means something different today from what it meant not long ago.

That being so, cultural anthropology is an effort to elucidate problematic relationships of meanings and symbols, a "natural history of signs and symbols, an ethnography of the vehicles of meaning."[3] The questions it asks are these:

> In a given set of meanings, which tangible symbols are employed to make those intangible meanings manifest, and how?
> Or from the symbols that circulate in a given culture, how can we reason back to uncover the meanings that move people, that people care about, that make the world real to them?
> How do symbols come to convey multiple different meanings?
> And how do meaning-and-symbol relationships change?

The name of this school of cultural anthropology is "hermeneutic," or for those of us who have trouble spelling that word and saying it, "interpretive."[4]

One quick illustration: Can science itself be polysemic? If so, how? Gary L. Downey's dissection of scientific meanings in American conflicts about nuclear power answers both those questions. Downey argues that in conflicts setting the nuclear industry against environmentalists, the former was typically seen to be a manifestation of science, so that environmentalists who disagreed with that industry were all too often diagnosed as hostile to science. But, says Downey, the environmentalists also included science in their ideologies. The various parties in a given controversy had substantially different understandings of science and thus different reasons for embracing science, which is to say that each party had its own meaning of science.[5]

The nuclear industry understood nuclear science in terms of the American philosophy of useful knowledge, which reduced science to technology and then celebrated that kind of science for making many people prosperous. Politically liberal environmentalists, usually from upper-middle-class backgrounds, understood science to be a valuable source of credible evidence. Science would help them demonstrate that the nuclear industry was unbalancing an implicit covenant of democratic culture when it diminished other peoples' enjoyment of the natural environment and that the industry did so without the benefit of a democratic decision-making process. Radical environmentalists likewise diagnosed science as valuable evidence, but they diagnosed technology as an evil force that created terrible social injustices. So there was a threefold appreciation of science "as a cultural source of authoritative knowledge about nature," yet each of these meanings was contingent on preexisting extrinsic political meanings: namely, those of prosperity, democratic process, and social justice, respectively.[6]

None of these parties was more friendly or more hostile to science than the others. Each integrated some scientific authority into its own ideology. The sum of this three-way balance was that none of the parties could convince the public that science corroborated its respective position while discrediting the others. "No decisive scientific conclusion about [nuclear] risk could be reached," writes Downey. "And so the battle continued as it began, a classificatory dispute among conflicting ideologies, with all sides invoking the authority of science, but none entirely successfully."[7]

OCCIDENTAL CULTURES

The interpretive school of cultural anthropology has traditionally been directed at non-Western cultures and has taught us much about their existential substance. More recently, however, this school has been turned around on itself so that now it is pointed at the Western cultures that produced it. Finally, we have an anthropology of occidental meanings and their symbols.

This anthropology-of-ourselves is still in a rudimentary stage and is often rattled by the bumps and potholes in the systems of meanings and symbols of Western cultures. After all, those occidental systems were seldom mapped in ethnographic detail before Western anthropologists began to run out of interpretive problems in the non-Western world. I do not mean that anthropologists have invented or reinvented occidental thought. I mean that anthropologists and others have only recently discovered that the systems of meanings and symbols by which the peoples of Western cultures try to figure out what life is all about are every bit as peculiar and problematic as those of other cultures.

A case in point of the challenges involved in studying occidental culture is the quantity of information that circulates within Western civilization. The amount of information available—data, texts, images, models, electronic memories—is more numerous than in any other culture in human history and in fact is now practically infinite. But this is far too much for any one individual, university, government, or interest group to digest. The humans of the Western cultures are choking on a surfeit of knowledge. The cultural meanings we depend on to make sense of all this information are failing us, both because these meanings cannot change as quickly as the information changes and because they cannot condense all of this information, or even most of it, into comprehensible systems of meanings and symbols.

The sharpest commentary on this condition comes from French sociologist Jean Baudrillard, who argues that relationships between meanings and symbols, even between tangible realities and visual representations of those realities, have been severely undermined in the modern cultures saturated by television and computers. These cultures, he suggests, consist mostly of images on images, which can now exist apart from the meanings and realities they were once meant to represent. In his books *Simulations* and *Selected Writings,* Baudrillard describes a "precession of simulacra," a trajectory of logic by which the Western world has moved from a culture in which signs and symbols were anchored in the meanings and realities that they supposedly represented to a culture in which signs and symbols have an autonomous life of their own.[8] For three millennia or so, the logic of representation that was central to Western thought (and that included hermeneutic theory, phenomenology, existentialism, Marxism, Freudianism, transubstantiation, consubstantiation, and hundreds of other -isms, -ologies, and -ations) presumed that there was a distinction between form and content or between tangible and ideal. It was supposed that there were some metaphysically essential realities and meanings, that we had images that referred to them, but that the fit between a metaphysical referent and its image was somewhat imperfect. If so, then the main tasks of Western thought were to measure the degree to which an image was faithful or unfaithful to its metaphysical referent, to say why it was unfaithful, and then to recommend the intellectual methods that would make the connection more faithful and thus less distorted.

Baudrillard takes those assumptions as his point of departure, and then leads his readers on a tour of the hermeneutic Gehenna of Western cultures in the late twentieth century.[9] The logic of representation—that an image reflects a reality—was succeeded by a suspicion that an image distorts a reality; and then by an accusation that an image conceals the absence of a reality.[10] The current stage of Western thinking about images and realities, says Baudrillard, is that of simulation: an image need not have any metaphysical relation to a reality.[11] "The spectre raised by simulation" is the "liquidation of all referentials": "Truth, reference, and objective causes have ceased to exist."[12] Elsewhere he calls this phenomenon "the implosion of meaning." "We are in a universe where there is more and more information, and less and less meaning."[13]

"Simulacra" is Baudrillard's term for symbols that have escaped reference to meanings or realities, and "hyperreality" is his name for their status in the occidental cultures of the late twentieth century. Images are anchored in other images and refer to other images; they do not need metaphysical referents. "There is no relationship between a system of meaning and a system of simulation."[14] Meanings and realities are passé.

Is this conclusion too grim and too dire to be true? Let us return to the fellow we met in chapter 1, the television actor in the white lab coat. Is he medical authority itself endorsing the product? No, of course he is not because medical authority is an intangible meaning and intangible meanings need tangible symbols. Is he a doctor, then, that is, a human reality who serves as a tangible symbol of medical authority? No, he is not, and in fact he plainly declares he is not a doctor. Then is he an actor who pretends to be a doctor, a symbol once removed from the human reality of a doctor and twice removed from the intangible meaning of medical authority? No, he is not that either. He is only an actor who candidly declares that he is only an actor.

If he is not a meaning, not a symbol once removed, and not a symbol twice removed, then what is he? Perhaps it is too grim and too dire to admit and maybe too awkward to pronounce, but he is a Baudrillardian simulacrum looking us in the eye and insulting our intelligence right in our own homes when we turn on our televisions. He is an image of medical authority, having none but the most preposterous reference to the meaning of medical authority or the reality of a physician. The reason this conjuring is possible is because, in Baudrillardian hyperreality, "there is no relationship between a system of meaning and a system of simulation."[15] The actor in the white lab coat can simulate medical authority without having to answer to the substantive meanings of medical authority, such as the simple assumption that an actor who plays a doctor is less credible than a doctor.

Can we specify which parts of the Western cultures are more hyperreal and which are more classically representational? Baudrillard directs his comments about the implosion of meaning more toward computer simulations ("matrices, memory banks, [and] command models") than to television.[16] To consider how television simulation has saturated the Western cultures, we can turn to argument 4 in Jerry Mander's book, *Four Arguments for the Elimination of Television:* "The technology of television predetermines the boundaries of its contents."[17] Mander demonstrates that "all television is real" in the sense that most viewers find all TV images equally authentic.[18] Following the logic of classical representation, viewers generally suppose that each television image is a faithful replication of a true event since television's visual grammar of nonfiction is more or less identical to its visual grammar of fiction. Docudramas, reenactments, and infomercials make fiction, fantasy, and fable interchangeable with nonfiction because on television all those others look like nonfiction. "The question of what is real and unreal," Mander writes, "is itself a new one, abstract and impossible to understand."[19] It happens frequently that viewers' perceptions of the world are seriously distorted by the selective imagery they see on television. This distortion has been noted anecdotally and measured statistically, revealing that the inability to distinguish reality from television correlates very closely with the number of hours that one watches television.[20]

Given that television is selective in the images it presents, to the point of seriously distorting human perception, then is there a pattern or structure to this distortion? The heart of Mander's argument 4 is that television's structural distortions are caused not by the conscious intentions of those who own the medium, but rather by unintended (yet unavoidable) technical features of the medium. Television, says Mander, has a signal-to-noise ratio that is especially problematic compared with that of other visual media, such as cinema or photography. Fine-grained visual images are lost, and foreground images blend into background images. To solve this problem, the medium of television selects images with little detail, stark background, and simple form, known collectively as "good television." Images that include or require nuance, subtlety, and context are poorly transmitted by the same medium. Inevitably, these are "bad television" in terms of the technology of electronically transmitting visual imagery.[21]

Close ups of peoples' faces are good television, whether in soap operas, sitcoms, sports events, talk shows, news reports, or science programs. So, too, "hate, fear, jealousy, winning, wanting, and violence" are the essense of "good television" because these kinds of content require fewer details, starker backgrounds, and more obvious forms than do other kinds of content.[22] Furthermore, competition between stations or between networks requires a large amount of visual razzle-dazzle to hold the viewer's attention and thus dissuade him or her from switching channels or, God forbid, turning off the television. Technical events such as cuts, pans, zooms, dissolves, and split screens occur about every six seconds during ordinary network television and much more often during commercials.[23] Again, this characteristic is not the intentional preference of those who own the medium but rather an artifact of television technology; this is the only successful way to organize visual images in a competitive market, for it holds the viewer's attention, almost to the point of hypnosis. But, says Mander, this visual razzle-dazzle is "technique as replacement of content" because the frantic pace of switching visual images makes it impossible for the viewer to follow any one thought for very long.[24]

So if all television is real, if this reality is selective because of technical constraints, and if television's selectivity includes simplistic visual imagery plus hyperactive image switching, then we have a good idea of the difference between the reality presented by good television and the residual reality—our lives outside of television—that makes for bad television. But even if we prefer our own bad-television lives to good television, Mander's observations still affirm that in the realm of television, Baudrillard's point is true about images existing independently of intangible meanings or tangible realities. Television images are real without reference to other realities. They are especially independent of nuance, subtlety, context, and other parts of the existential substance of human culture that anthropologists call "meaning." Thus, we can find Baudrillardian hyperreality at its worst in television. When the Western cultures, particularly American culture, are overly influenced by this medium, then the classic epistemology of representation, which makes hermeneutics worth pursuing, is eclipsed by the new antiepistemology of simulation, which makes hermeneutics maddening.

The lessons we can draw from Geertz and Baudrillard, with a dash of Mander, are these:

1. Human culture is problematic because symbols are polysemic. Different kinds of people derive different meanings from the same symbols.
2. Culture is further complicated by changes in the relations of meanings and symbols.
3. The representational logic of the Western cultures is in a crisis of hyperreality because of the rise of simulation. Symbols and images often refer only to other images and symbols, in which case intangible meaning and tangible reality are irrelevant.
4. The disarticulation of images and symbols from meanings and realities is especially acute in the case of television and in those parts of the Western cultures that are influenced by television.

AN ANTHROPOLOGY OF SCIENCE
IN AMERICAN CULTURE

In the American style for making decisions about scientific issues, called "democratic science," multiple parties participate in shaping decisions. Decisions might be made directly, as through referenda, or indirectly, as through informal processes of consensus or through multilayered processes of checks and balances. Regardless, nonscientists play important roles along with scientists. Just as there are different kinds of scientists with different kinds of values, so the same can be said of nonscientists. If we refer to the beliefs, philosophies, ideologies, and values of these various parties as meanings, and if people need symbols to understand, communicate, and act on their respective meanings, then polysemic symbols will inevitably complicate democratic science. Within any given episode of democratic science, there can be many different understandings of science and its implications for our lives.

Those understandings are the stuff of interpretive anthropology because they are problematic relationships between meanings and symbols. They include instances in which the Protestant model of science is eclipsed by the scientific research ethos, the moral autonomy of science collapses in an age of moral cynicism and financial limitations, or each of three different parties in nuclear controversies can credibly maintain three different visions of science.

In the more severe examples of this problem, the meanings and realities of science are passing into Baudrillardian hyperreality, where they are turned to vapor and replaced by images grounded in nothing but other images. Such is the case when an actor who says he is not a doctor is an effective simulacrum for the authority of medical science, when the tobacco lobby can turn its own long-held standards of scientific proof upside down and inside out but still hold the exact same position on the risks of secondhand smoke, and when a zoologist motivates tens of thousands by predicting a massive earthquake on the basis of blatantly specious reasoning.

This kind of mischief with images is the business of the conjurer: to fashion an ersatz semblance of something using only gimmicks and sleight of hand. The tools of the trade could be some smoke, some mirrors, and a trapdoor if the object is to conjure an apparition of a ghost. But they could also be scientific credentials, technical terms, or standards of scientific proof if the task at hand is to conjure science.

Finally, we should consider Mander's litany of epistemological biases in TV reality and from that litany draw an important insight about the science-television relationship. His litany includes these items:

- "Superficiality is easier [to present] than depth."
- "The medium cannot deal with ambiguity, subtlety, and diversity."
- "The bizarre always gets more attention on television than the usual."
- "Death is easier [to transmit] than life [because] it is specific, focused, highlighted, fixed, resolved, and has meaning aside from context."[25]

These features of television are unremarkable when the content of science is simplistic, superficial, unambiguous, bizarre, or macabre. But when science has interesting substance, then the insight we derive from Mander is that good science makes bad television. The intellectual depth and value of scientific thought are inversely related to television's ability to communicate such content. If we value science, we should fall to our knees and say this prayer: God preserve us from science on television.

So to return to the more general discussion of science in American life, I offer some simple guidelines for an interpretive anthropology. First, nonscientists' meanings of science are just as germane as scientists'. This guideline does not suggest that either are necessarily good science, good for science, or anchored in any kind of scientific knowledge or reasoning. It only indicates that the process of figuring out what science means is open to many. In any given dispute, different parties are welcome to put forth very different kinds of meanings about science. Democratic science is politically gracious and hermeneutically promiscuous.

A related point is that in democratic science the meanings and symbols of science may be entirely unconnected to either the substantive content of scientific knowledge or the logical structure of scientific reasoning. Of course, the various meanings of science found in democratic science have undeniable existential value, but there is no requirement that this value has to articulate with, or be relevant to, scientific knowledge or reasoning. Such value might be downright contrary to those standards, but this does not exclude it from democratic science.

To appreciate this gap between the substance of science and the democratic meanings of science, we can recall that most of our schoolchildren are miserably uneducated in science, that this misery increases as they advance through our schools, and that landslide majorities of our adult American population are scientifically illiterate. None of these conditions diminishes the power or authority of scientific symbols. The God of the Old Testament is still our paradigm for science, so the hermeneutics of fear, mystery, and awe shape the role of science in American life.

Next we have to ask awkward questions. If the popular symbols of science are available to be borrowed, stolen, distorted, and manipulated by causes and ideologies unconnected to the substance of science, then what are the nonscientific meanings of science that are made manifest by the symbols of science? *Why* do people conjure science? Given that the symbols of science truly have the power to enhance commodities, policies, and ideologies, what are the meanings being enhanced if they are not science?

Finally, we have to question the cultural dynamics of science in American life. If the popular symbols of science and the meanings they manifest do not have to be grounded in the intellectual content of science, then how do those symbols become separated from the content of science and then associated with nonscientific meanings? How is scientific credibility separated from science so that it gives credibility to meanings that have nothing to do with science? *How* is science conjured?

So we have a multilayered headache of science, symbols, and meanings, but we also have a program of interpretive anthropology for understanding this headache (not for curing it, only for understanding it). Luckily, this anthropology of science has its own Magna Carta, a founding document that defines principles and steers us toward a constructive program of research. Ironically, its author is not an anthropologist but rather a historian, Charles E. Rosenberg. His 1966 essay "Science in American Social Thought" acknowledges that the role of science in this society includes the professional values and attitudes of scientists but then emphasizes that this role is hardly limited to those factors. Far more salient, says Rosenberg, is the custom of looting science for images and metaphors to illustrate bourgeois morality. When the nervous system is explained through comparison to a telegraph company, when emotional moderation is justified in terms of the second law of thermodynamics, or when forensic psychiatry can be interpreted to corroborate both liberal and conservative social theory, then this tells us much about extrascientific matters such as telegraph companies, emotional moderation, liberalism, and conservatism.[26]

Such comparison, justification, and interpretation tell us next to nothing, however, about the respective sciences of neurology, thermodynamics, or psychiatry, except that their scientific vocabularies can be expropriated for purposes that have nothing to do with those fields.[27] Or as an anthropologist might say, scientific symbols are available to express nonscientific meanings. As Rosenberg remarks, "There is a logic here, arbitrary and makeshift as these 'scientific' analogies may seem. It is to be found, not in their particular scientific content, but in their social function. We must look, not to the internal coherence of the [scientific] ideas appropriated, but at their external logic— that is, their social purpose."[28]

It would be reasonable to presume that this feature of science, that it can easily be used to convey nonscientific meaning, would undermine its credibility. But this is not the case. That feature has done nothing to diminish the rise of scientific respectability: "One of the most important developments in the relationship between science and American social thought has been the increasing emotional relevance of science, its growing role as an absolute [authority] able to justify and motivate individual action."[29] Science is believed to be objective, nonpartisan, and able to fix the worst of our social problems (and without upsetting our social structure!), even while the intellectual content of scientific knowledge and reasoning is not particularly relevant to this power of science.

To summarize this anthropology of science:

1 Science is widely thought to have a plenary authority to define reality, even though this power seems mysterious (science in an Old Testament style).

2. At the same time, this form of authority is available to numerous parties on a more or less equal basis, which is to say that the business of defining science and its implications is open to all (democratic science).

3. Thus, there is no requirement that the various competing claims

about science and its implications have to be constrained by standards of scientific knowledge or anchored in scientific reasoning.

4. As a result, the plenary authority of science can be invoked to endorse or enhance ideologies, commodities, and policies, regardless of whether they are grounded in science, by deploying the popular symbols of science.

5. Interpretive anthropology offers a program for understanding how the symbols of science become severed from the substance of science and then reattached to other meanings; this program is based on Geertz's discussion of meanings and symbols, Baudrillard's analysis of reality and simulation, and Rosenberg's commentary on science and American social thought.

Now let us see if my approach works. In the next five chapters I present five episodes of science in American life, each of them involving a different problem of scientific symbols and cultural meanings. Together they indicate the scope of the grand problem: the cultural life of these symbols is such that they can be attached to almost any sort of meaning.

I offer one caveat. In these case studies it may seem that I am passing judgment on good science versus bad science or that I try to damn pseudoscience by holding it up against true science. But that is not what I want to do. When I discover that some symbols of science have become attached to various cultural meanings, this implies that they ought to be attached to science instead. That kind of reference back to science is unavoidable. But in these episodes, the hermeneutics of meanings and symbols is much more important than the metaphysics of good science versus bad.

Thus, chapter 5 is not a textbook account of the science of fluoridation. Rather, it is a story about the fear of losing one's soul to impersonal institutions. When the policy of fluoridating water was implicated in that fear, this story also became a tale of scientific symbols and cultural meanings. Remember that its true worth is hermeneutic, not metaphysical. The same goes for the other four chapters in part 3. Each asks the same two questions: What meanings are invested in this thought about science? And how are the symbols of science attached to those meanings?

PART THREE

Episodes

CHAPTER FIVE

■ ■ ■

Soul-Snatching

If ever science was subjected to cultural meaning, then the case of fluoridation was the granddaddy of this family of phenomena. The fluoridation controversies, as a problem of understanding and misunderstanding science and values, had their origins in the cultural and political naïveté of the public health officials who advocated a policy of fluoridating public supplies of drinking water. Those officials constructed a remarkably simple argument: fluoridation was good for you because epidemiology, dentistry, and biochemistry said so, in which case the officials needed only to proclaim that view and then institute it. But this argument was, at best, condescending to citizens, who knew little or nothing of the scientific basis of fluoridation. At worst, it was downright frightening, for it meant that unknown bureaucrats would require us to ingest chemicals about which we knew little.

Subsequently, a counterargument arose according to which flouridation was an evil plot by faceless bureaucrats to steal your soul. If true, then every act of opposition, including opposition to the program's scientific premises, was a heroic act of existential virtue. For at least the first decade and a half of the fluoridation controversies, from 1950 through 1966, the argument against fluoridation prevailed in 59.4 percent of 952 referenda on this question.[1]

To understand this intermingling of science and meaning, I present a brief history of the fluoridation controversies. I then identify the main cultural themes of American life in the 1950s that animated antifluoridation sentiment. Following that, I show how certain symbols of science served the cause of the antifluoridationists, even while the advocates of fluoridation believed that science served only themselves.

A SHORT HISTORY OF FLUORIDATION

Dr. Frederick McKay, a dentist in Colorado, noticed in 1901 that many of his patients exhibited mottling, a minor cosmetic effect in which tiny spots of dull white appeared on teeth that should have been uniformly shiny white. As it turned out, mottling was a regional phenomenon; colloquial names like "Texas Teeth" and "Colorado Brown Teeth" referred to its more severe forms, in which teeth were noticeably discolored. By 1916, McKay had identified fluoride, which occurred naturally in the drinking water of some areas, as the source of mottling. The more fluoride there was in the water, the more severe was the mottling. Hence, severe mottling was called fluorosis.[2]

McKay and others also noticed that the less severe levels of mottling were closely associated with good dental health, that is, fewer cavities and stronger teeth. In 1931 epidemiologists confirmed that this mottling, too, had its source in naturally occurring fluoride. The landmark case study was that of Minonk, Illinois, where fluoride occurred naturally in the drinking water at 2.5 parts per million (ppm). Children raised in Minonk had much less tooth decay than children who had moved there after their tooth development had been completed elsewhere. The U.S. Public Health Service (USPHS) then studied thirteen communities in five states and concluded that more fluoride resulted in less tooth decay. This result was corroborated in twelve other countries.[3]

The U.S. Public Health Service began four case-control studies in 1945 to test the hypothesis that if a community's drinking water was artificially fluoridated at 1.0 ppm, then this would greatly improve children's dental health but without causing mottling or any other side effects. (The threshold for minor mottling is approximately 2.5 ppm.)[4] In New York, Michigan, Illinois, and Ontario, respectively, one community each received artificial fluoridation and a comparable community served as the control, receiving none, whether naturally or artificially. The study was intended to consume ten years, but when the USPHS discovered reductions in children's cavities of 50 percent or more within five years in the case-study communities, it concluded that artificial fluoridation was a great success. In 1950 the USPHS recommended that communities without naturally occurring fluoride artificially add it to their public water supplies at a concentration of 1.0 ppm. Organizations endorsing this policy included the American Dental

Association, the American Medical Association, the American Association of Public Health Dentists, and the National Research Council.[5]

Fluoride could also be delivered via tablets and food additives, but these methods were very imperfect because they depended on discipline, convenience, cost, and other behavioral variables. By contrast, it was extremely simple and inexpensive to fluoridate a community's drinking water, which then reached almost everyone, regardless of behavioral differences.[6]

Thousands of communities adopted the Public Health Service's recommendations and added fluoride to their water, but in numerous cases there were vehement reactions against this practice. The typical pattern was for a public health department to recommend fluoridation to the town or city council on the basis of the USPHS recommendation, along with the endorsements of other authorities. There would be little or no public interest at the time of the decision, but then an angry *anti*fluoridation movement would arise at about the time that the policy was implemented, that is, when the public drinking water was actually affected. The most common strategy of the antifluoridationists was to call for a referendum on this practice. There were 952 such referenda between 1950 and 1966; in 566 of them the opponents of fluoridation won.[7]

One of the useful aspects of a referendum is that it quantifies sentiment, which is to say that its results can be correlated with other data. As a matter of interest politics, the voters most favorable to fluoridation were young parents with children under twelve, who would benefit most from fluoride, whereas the opponents were older, either childless or with grown children, who would benefit least. In socioeconomic terms, the advocates generally had completed higher levels of education, and had higher incomes, than the opponents. The former were often professionals and managers, while the latter more likely had working-class and lower-middle-class occupations. Finally, the advocates possessed a confidence that they could affect political matters, whereas the antifluoridation voters tended to feel helpless or powerless in that regard. This last point is the most important of all, for reasons that will unfold as we consider the cultural climate of the fluoridation referenda.[8]

The referendum results distressed the social scientists studying the fluoridation controversy. Bernard and Judith Mausner, for example, labeled antifluoridationist views "the anti-scientific attitude."[9] On the basis of interviews, census data, and other information, a group of researchers interpreted those results in terms of a model embracing three issues: (1) *effectiveness* (i.e., does fluoridation really accomplish what its advocates contend?); (2) *safety* (what are the side effects, and how dangerous are they?); and (3) *individual rights* (is fluoridation a governmental invasion into the private life of the individual?).

The first issue was the least problematic. Epidemiological studies from earlier in the century were sufficiently convincing that opponents of fluoridation seldom challenged them directly. Instead, opponents implicitly conceded that fluoride was effective but then argued that dental health was not important enough to justify universal measures since tooth decay was neither contagious nor fatal.[10]

The second issue was more complicated. Opponents said that fluoride had serious toxic side effects, for example, headaches, fatigue, fainting, and painful joints. They pointed to widespread reports of those events and to goldfish dying in fluoridated water. In addition, opponents reminded the public that sodium fluoride was a rat poison and that fluorine was a component of nerve gas. The profluoridationists answered that the two forms of fluoride added to drinking water (calcium fluoride and sodium aluminum fluoride) were quite different from those two poisons.[11] While profluoridationists conceded that almost any substance can have a toxic effect in enormous quantities, they argued that a substance like fluoride can also be perfectly safe in small doses.[12] Profluoridationists described the threshold of toxicity for fluoride, at 1.0 ppm, as the amount of fluoride in fifty bathtubs of water consumed at one time.[13] If so, then this threshold would be impossible to reach. The would-be sufferer would destroy his or her stomach and kidneys long before fluoride could do any damage. Furthermore, seafood typically contained fluoride at 5.0 to 15.0 ppm; tea leaves, at 75.0 to 100.0 ppm. This substance was "omnipresent" in all the foods from plant or animal sources that people consumed.[14] Nevertheless, public health authorities could not give assurances of 100 percent certainty that no one would have an adverse reaction.

The last of the three issues was especially intractable. Public health officials believed they had a responsibility to improve the dental health of children, especially if fluoridation was effective, safe, and inexpensive. The other side felt strongly that fluoridating someone's drinking water amounted to an impersonal bureaucracy invading the most private part of our lives, that is, our bodies, by "pour[ing] chemicals indiscriminately down the throats of those who need dentistry and those who don't."[15]

The richest exploration of this issue was Arnold Green's article "The Ideology of the Anti-Fluoridation Leaders," wherein the author argued that this ideology concentrated numerous forms of alienation, social fears, and miscellaneous anxieties. "The fluoridation controversy," he wrote, is "a surrogate issue" for other concerns, such as that the modern world would "smother personal identity in a homogeneous mass."[16]

A series of empirical reports accepted this three-issue model. Collectively the reports implied, to one degree or another, that fluoridation was effective (thus resolving the first of the three issues) and that it was safe (settling the second issue), in which case the main problem was to explain why so many people could not accept what science had demonstrated about safety and effectiveness. The reports' answer lay in the third issue: if a citizen worried about dehumanization, this warped his or her ability to think clearly about the scientific basis of the first two issues.[17] The existential problem of losing one's identity to impersonal forces, it seemed, could not be legitimately connected to genuine scientific questions. Instead, the three-issue model treated the third issue, the matter of cultural meanings, as a rude and spurious intrusion into the scientific discussion of fluoridation.

As Mausner and Mausner pointed out, it was easy for voters to appreciate the argument that fluoridation robbed us of our individual freedom because this argument was grounded in certain common cultural values.[18] Consequently, opposition to fluoridation has persisted well beyond the halcyon days of daily headlines in the 1950s. Anti-fluoridation sentiment became institutionalized in an organization called the National Health Federation.[19] From this and similar sources came accusations that fluoride caused cancer, Down's syndrome, cardiovascular disease, and even AIDS.[20] In response, Consumers Union published a two-part rebuttal and exposé in 1978, blasting the National Health Federation for being linked to right-wing extremists such as the John Birch Society and accusing the federation of using "six ways to mislead the public," that is, of systematically distorting scientific evidence.[21]

Nevertheless, the union's critique hardly caused opposition to fluoride to evaporate, for a trio of scholarly articles published in 1988 forcefully renewed the challenge to fluoridation policies. The most influential was Bette Hileman's review in *Chemical and Engineering News*, gathering together numerous fears, allegations, and warnings about the possible toxic consequences of fluoride. Old arguments about dental fluorosis, with lots of new data, and new arguments about cancer, for example, made this a most disturbing piece to read. When Hileman charged that advocates of fluoridation had suppressed damning information about the toxicity of fluoride, this seemed ominous indeed.[22] At the very least, the reader could quickly agree with Hileman's contention that more research should be done on problems such as carcinogenicity.

And yet for all the urgency and passion, there was something about fluoridation missing at the core of this article. Hileman was aggressively skeptical about the practice of fluoridation, and she used many hypotheses very effectively to challenge its wisdom. But she never charged that fluoridation was surely poisonous or even that it was probably poisonous. Instead, her style was to say repeatedly that objections had been raised, that the objections were not conclusive, and that more research should be done to address these objections. She raised numerous very serious issues but without resolving them. In lieu of a firm stand on empirical issues, the author subverted support for fluoridation by creating an ominous tone of uncertainty and suspicion.

The second of these 1988 articles addressed one specific problem, a hypothetical "critical mass" of fluoride in which fluoridated drinking water was combined with that from other sources such that the total of all fluoride could reach toxic levels. The writer, Geoffrey Smith, easily agreed that fluoride in drinking water was very effective at reducing cavities; but, he contended, there was so much additional fluoride in industrial waste and pesticides, not to mention toothpastes, mouthwashes, and food additives, that all these sources together might raise levels well above the threshold for toxicity. He indicated, for example, that people living in areas without fluoridated drinking water sometimes exhibited the effects of fluoridation (reduced cavities), presumably because of these many other sources. In that case, Smith asked, "if people in unfluoridated areas are receiving 'sufficient' fluoride, then are some people in fluoridated areas receiving too much?"[23]

In a way this article was conciliatory, for it accepted the central premise of the fluoridationists: that fluoride was effective. But Smith, too, subverted the argument for fluoridation, not exactly by declaring that toxic levels had been reached, but rather by suggesting strongly that this *might* have happened or *might* do so in the near future. At one time fluoride was good, but now it is—or rather could be—too much of a good thing. Smith reiterated that things were "not fully understood," "not known with any certainty," and were "yet to be resolved." Evidence was "conflicting and inconclusive"; "further studies . . . are needed"; "new evidence may emerge."[24] His overall strategy was the same as Hileman's. He did not need to assert his own argument conclusively, only arouse a disturbing sense of uncertainty, to effectively challenge the practice of fluoridating drinking water.

Brian Martin, the third author in 1988, diagnosed the fluoridation controversy as a struggle for power and control. In a sharp departure from previous arguments for and against fluoridation that had appealed to empirical evidence and scientific authority, Martin set aside scientific evidence and suggested instead that the issue of fluoridation be considered an amoral contest to control certain resources (professional associations, scientific journals) and whatever power came with those resources. From this view, epidemiologists, dentists, and biochemists endorsed fluoridation for reasons that had nothing to do with the scientific value of fluoridation. On the contrary, "claims by scientists . . . [should be treated] as ploys in a social struggle in which it is advantageous to be seen above the struggle."[25] Scientific judgment was likewise irrelevant to the institutional endorsements of fluoridation by professional associations: "It is the control over political resources associated with the dental and medical professions which gives rise to the major asymmetry in the fluoridation debate."[26]

Martin's special contribution was to open up a whole new intellectual front for antifluoridation sentiment. He drew on a relatively new school of thought, the sociology of scientific knowledge, which defined scientific thought as a value-laden creation produced through social negotiation. This definition, of course, suggested both that the empirical foundations of scientific knowledge were overrated and that science was more of a social conflict to seize power than a disinterested search for the truth about nature. Martin further elaborated on this approach in a 1989 sociology article.[27] The same view appeared even more bluntly in his book on fluoridation, published in 1991, wherein he asserted that "power is involved in all aspects of the practice of science, even in the daily processes by which scientists make decisions about what is valid knowledge," and that "it is impossible to separate the scientific and power dimensions of the fluoridation issue."[28]

Close to the surface of Martin's approach was a grand tautology: the reason one side controlled the debate was because this debate was about control. One might have expected that feature to have scorched both sides equally, but this was not so. Martin was occasionally critical of the antifluoridationists, but he pointed out that relativism like his would deliver a greater sting to the advocates.[29] After all, the advocates of fluoridation believed that their strong suit was the empirical evidence regarding the effectiveness and safety of fluoridation. If so, then a sociology skeptical of empirical scientific knowledge would take out the heart of their cause and replace it with a view that both sides were morally equivalent in a political struggle for power and control.

And so Martin argued, in his 1988 article, his 1989 article, and his 1991 book, that those who endorsed fluoridation had not examined either the scientific or ethical issues carefully.[30] Their organization endorsements were factually suspect, he implied.[31] In both articles and in the book, Martin presented the grievances of the antifluoridationists very sympathetically, but he tainted those of the fluoridationists with a thick measure of cynicism. Although it is hard to gauge the effect of an approach that denies a place for science in a scientific controversy, the effect, if any, of Martin's work must have been to discredit the advocates of fluoridation.

One last problem: Martin had located the great struggle for power only within professional organizations such as the American Dental Association. There, he declared, the profluoridation forces had won that struggle since those organizations had endorsed the policy of fluoridating public supplies of drinking water. But the question of fluoridation was also pursued in thousands of American communities, often by means of a referendum. The parties supposedly in control of political resources within the professional associations were the losers in six out of ten of those referenda, which means either that their power was not very powerful or that Martin's definition of the location of power was extremely narrow.

When a 1989 memo within the Environmental Protection Agency raised the possibility that fluoride had caused osteosarcoma in rats, both *Science* and *Newsweek* reported the memo in detail, and they also revisited the argument that fluoride in sources such as toothpaste was making drinking-water fluoride redundant.[32] The EPA responded by giving the National Research Council (NRC) of the National Academy of Sciences a mandate to review the osteosarcoma issue, plus all other suspicions of toxicity. The NRC formed a subcommittee on fluoride, which then addressed fluorosis, gastrointestinal effects, carcinogenicity, genotoxicity, and other questions.

The data on carcinogenicity in rats were equivocal at best and could not be replicated, even at higher doses, said the subcommittee report. As to fluorosis, that was a well-known problem at extremely high levels (8.0 ppm), according to the report, but there was no cause for alarm at 4.0 ppm or less. All in all, the NRC report discredited each charge of toxicity, at least as much as each could be discredited given the knowledge available at that time.[33]

The cultural issues, however, were not quite so tractable. Academic advocates of fluoridation, especially Mausner and Mausner, Benjamin Paul, and Harvey Sapolsky, accounted for the success of the antifluoridation forces by separating the scientific issues from the cultural meanings. Science affirmed that fluoridation was beneficial, they said or implied, and that it had no serious side effects. But too many people believed the worst about fluoridation because their emotional fears of a dehumanizing bureaucracy overwhelmed their faith in scientific authority.

Both of those statements describe a *part* of the American experience with fluoridation, but that overall analysis is a little too neat in the way it separates the scientific issues from the cultural ones. For example, if the fluoridationists were scientific and the antifluoridationists were emotional, then how could the latter have prevailed so often in a culture that ordinarily worships science as the source of prosperity and happiness?

A better approach is to reject the science-versus-emotion model and recognize instead that cultural meanings enveloped the scientific issues. Scientists' credentials, organizational endorsements, epidemiological studies, and interpretations of their results were subjected to cultural processes such that there was no objective voice of pure science. In that case, the problem of the fluoridation controversies is to understand the cultural meanings that framed this experience and to identify the cultural processes by which science was subjected to those forces.

CULTURAL MEANINGS IN THE
FLUORIDATION DISPUTES

Existential worries about one's individual uniqueness are both common and eternal, but they are seldom as painful as they were in the United States from the late 1940s to the mid-1960s, when the rise of large impersonal bureaucracies seemed especially threatening. During World War II, military service subjected millions of Americans to its standardized impersonal culture and even intentionally broke down their individual personalities (temporarily!) during basic training. After the war, giant corporations such as IBM and General Motors absorbed many of these people and required much more conformity than most Americans were comfortable with. In the person of Charles E. Wilson, the president of General Motors was interchangable with the secretary of defense.

Two of Arthur Miller's plays, *The Crucible* and *An Enemy of the People,* gave voice to the fear that conformity was equivalent to mob psychology and to the hope that heroes would resist it. Sloane Wilson's novel *The Man in the Gray Flannel Suit* told the story of a decent man being swallowed up by an impersonal corporation. David Riesman's sociology textbook *The Lonely Crowd* supported that theme with a theory about conflicts between the individual and society. *The Organization Man*, by W. H. White Jr., described how corporations enforced conformity through hiring, promotion, and the misuse of standardized personality tests. Ordinarily one assumed that corporations succeeded by rewarding initiative, leadership, and intelligence; but, said White, they only encouraged people to be statistically normal by subjecting employees to standardized tests. To help his readers with this dilemma—how to be an individual when your company wants you to be a drone—he added an appendix titled "How to Cheat on Personality Tests." Behind each test was a theory about a statistically normal personality. If the employee could infer the norm for a given test, then he or she could pass by *pretending* to be statistically normal.[34]

The material pleasures of consumer culture aggravated the anxiety that each of us was losing his or her individuality. The United States was more prosperous and more comfortable than any other nation in history, but this prosperity owed much to mass production. If one measured happiness in terms of material possessions (homes, cars, appliances, furniture), then the more successful one was, the more one possessed the same things that many others had.[35] Levittown, the instantly created New York suburb made of mass-produced homes, was a case in point: prosperity was made possible by homogeneity.

The "Davey Crockett" series on *The Walt Disney Show* was an electrifying success because the title character was a dramatic symbol of rugged individualism. No danger here that the man in the coonskin cap would succumb to consumer comforts or statistical norms. But when little boys tried to become rugged individuals like Davey, they began by wearing mass-produced coonskin caps, with the result that all these little would-be rugged individuals looked alike.

When we consider how acute were these cultural themes of individualism versus impersonal forces, then we see that the cold war fear of the Soviets was at least as much an existential panic as a security issue. If the Soviets conquered us, whether by violence or subterfuge, the worst consequence of all would be that we would become equally dreary, identical zombies. Indeed, some U.S. prisoners returning from the Korean War horrified the nation by exhibiting the effects of brainwashing, in which sophisticated psychological techniques could truly steal a person's emotions, virtues, and individuality.

Consider the case of Herbert Philbrick, author of *I Led Three Lives*. He seemed to be a normal guy, but he was really a communist spy. When you accepted that he was a communist spy, you learned he was really an informant for the Federal Bureau of Investigation. He succeeded as an F.B.I. informant, but he was really a normal guy. What lessons could one learn from Herbert Philbrick's story? Soviet spies looked like us, dressed like us, and acted like us. You could not be sure that someone you knew well was not a Soviet agent or even that you were not being manipulated by the Soviets.

Clinical progress in psychiatry and psychology contributed to the feeling that the personality was dangerously fragile. Battle fatigue, hypnosis, amnesia, personality disintegration, multiple personality disorder—as these phenomena were increasingly subjected to medical treatment, then one's personal problems, or a family's private business, became the stuff of very public conversation through films such as *The Three Faces of Eve*.

Similarly, public interest in Freudian thought led to simplistic and reductionist adages. Life was a series of identity crises. Deep down, everything was about sex. Each of us was secretly tormented by conflicting forces. The landscape of psychodynamics was a very dangerous terrain wherein each of us was buffeted by superhuman powers. These powers were subconscious, so one could be having a terrible identity crisis but not even realize it. The only hope was to turn to a professional therapist—a stranger—for explanations. In these circumstances, the man or woman with enough self-confidence to be happy and well adjusted was rare—also pathetically deluded, according to the usual psychological paradigms.

The films of that age affirmed this notion. In the films of the 1930s, contends Paul Jensen, virtue was clear, villains obvious, solutions simple, and most people good. But postwar films thrived on pessimism, guilt, helplessness, manipulation, and a fear "of being deprived of identity, individuality, and independency by some outside, infiltrating force."[36] Our confidence in ourselves—indeed, even our knowledge of ourselves—was undermined when "all sorts of guilt turned up on the screen: self-guilt, assumed guilt, generalized guilt, uncertainty of guilt, guilt by association, and mistaken guilt based on circumstantial evidence."[37] Psychiatrists revealed these flaws in us but could not help us because the psychiatrists in these films were often crazy. Authorities ought to have protected us from evil forces, but frequently the authorities were agents of evil forces.

In the minds of many people, there was a direct link between these endless rounds of personality crises and one's unpleasant experiences with large impersonal bureaucracies. The latter caused the former because bureaucracies were evil conspiracies for *intentionally* destroying our individuality. Don Siegel's 1956 film *The Invasion of the Body Snatchers* brilliantly captured that spirit by suggesting a series of extremely disturbing dangers. A person could not trust friends, neighbors, even close relatives because people were not who they seemed to be. A person could not even trust himself or herself because the personality was so brittle that he or she might suddenly become a different person. And then manipulating these weaknesses was an evil conspiracy that wore the face of trustworthy authority but that betrayed that trust. Its agents were faceless, impersonal, and anonymous but nevertheless able to snatch souls. Finally, the only form of protection from this monstrous threat was to be ever vigilant. In other words, constantly paranoid.

Given those possibilities, the title of Siegel's film was slightly misleading. The evil conspiracy snatched its victims' bodies, but it generously replaced them with faithful replicas. More to the point, it snatched Americans' souls—their emotions, their virtues, their individuality—and replaced them with nothing.

The practice of fluoridating drinking water thus arose at the worst possible moment. In retrospect it is easy to see why many Americans felt that fluoridation was another in a series of attempts to snatch our souls. Antifluoridationists often believed they were facing a gigantic evil conspiracy embracing faceless scientists, impersonal scientific organizations, the Aluminum Company of America, the American Dental Association, and the U.S. Public Health Service.[38] Not surprisingly, the antifluoridationists were often people with "a sense of powerlessness [who] seek ways of attacking people whom they perceive as powerful."[39] John Kirscht added that the antifluoridationists generally felt pessimistic, even helpless, about a series of problems, and William Gamson gave qualified approval to the hypothesis that antifluoridation sentiment correlated with an inability to cope with the world.[40] That being so, fluoridation could only be "an infringement of individual rights," an attempt "to smother personal identity in a homogeneous mass," "an outrageous example" of "discourag[ing] the exercise of individual responsibility."[41] To oppose it was obviously "an act of moral resistance."[42]

Regardless of other developments in the fluoridation controversy, that sentiment is still durable. In February 1990, conservative columnist James J. Kilpatrick reminded his readers that "the deeper issue [i.e., deeper than the medical issues] is now, and always has been, the issue of personal freedom. Whatever may be said for fluoridation as a matter of public health, the program is a patent invasion of private rights—specifically, the right of each individual to control the medicine he takes."[43] With a colorful flourish, he added that "if the choice is between losing a bicuspid or losing a freedom, let the bicuspid go."[44]

So strong was this sense of individual freedom that it had profound consequences for the second issue, that of safety. If one accepted that large impersonal bureaucracies intentionally tried to destroy our individuality, then the supposed toxicity of fluoride was not merely an accidental side effect. In fact, it was a diabolical weapon, a poison known to be a poison and used as such. Arnold Green traced a certain chain of logic in antifluoridation thought: (1) poison presumes a poisoner, that is, an evil agent who has malicious intentions (which is to say that bureaucrats are trying to eradicate our individuality); (2)

an evil agent will obviously use deception and disguise to achieve his or her goals; (3) the effect of poisoning is to put the victim under the control of the poisoner; and (4) the victim cannot locate the source of poison (because the poisoner operates from behind the cover of a faceless impersonal bureaucracy).[45]

The accusation that fluoride was poison became considerably more plausible when framed by the issue of personal freedom versus impersonal bureaucracy. According to Green's interpretation, "People most sensitive and responsive to the poison symbolism feel that in some other crucial areas of life, their autonomy and integrity as individuals are under severe attack. They sense something conspiratorial in the assault upon them."[46]

This kind of sensitivity also meant that the issue of effectiveness could no longer be resolved empirically, for it had become a moral question instead and a very polarized moral question at that. Either the antifluoridationists were paranoid because they could not handle the complexities of twentieth-century life, or the advocates of fluoridation were agents of some evil force, whether they knew it or not.

THE CULTURAL DYNAMICS OF SCIENCE

What about science? Were those fears of losing one's individual identity so strong that they swept away the scientific knowledge supporting fluoridation and drowned out the scientific authorities who advocated it? Actually, something more subtle happened. In lieu of a head-on collision between fear and scientific knowledge, the antifluoridation ideology neutralized profluoridation science by subjecting it to a pair of cultural processes, which I call the "pseudosymmetry of scientific authority" and the "heavy weight of scientific uncertainty."

During the referendum campaign in Northampton, Massachusetts, the most important antifluoridation leader was a professional chemist with solid scientific credentials. Local antifluoridationists readily credited his scientific authority, but they "overwhelmingly refused to accept . . . scientific organizations as the best authorities on fluoridation. . . . The anti-fluoridation voters on the whole seemed to be more impressed by the few deviant scientists and professional people who opposed fluoridation than by the organized medical and scientific groups that favored it."[47] In a similar case, the 1953 campaign in Cambridge, Massachusetts, one of the most influential antifluoridationists was a local physician who frequently challenged the city's health commissioner, often debating him at public meetings.[48]

At the national level, John Lear's articles in the *Saturday Review,* where Lear's title was "science editor," were extremely influential because the magazine was highbrow, hardly vulnerable to suspicions of being a platform for right-wing hysteria.[49] But Lear based his vehement critique of fluoridation on only two scientific articles, as if these two were equivalent to the many scientific articles embracing fluoridation.

Robert Rodale's 1961 letter to *Science* summarized the argument that scientific authority was about equally divided on the question of fluoridation:

> It is true, of course, that the Public Health Service and the American Dental Association are on the side of fluoridation, but that does not mean that there are not very reputable and capable scientists who are opposed to fluoridation and who have produced evidence indicating that fluoridation is a potentially harmful practice. The voter in a fluoridation election, therefore, is put in the position of choosing between two branches of scientific thought.[50]

Meanwhile, advocates of fluoridation, especially dentists, too often hesitated to endorse fluoridation enthusiastically, perhaps because they underestimated the opposition. The unintended result of this hesitancy was that it abetted the impression that scientific experts were truly divided about evenly, hence the pseudosymmetry of scientific authority.[51] Thus, Martin and others observe that "even a few dissenting scientists, if they are willing to speak out . . . have a political impact much larger than is suggested by their isolated position."[52]

This phenomenon, that a handful of scientific authorities had as much credibility as many, was especially effective in referendum campaigns. To fluoridate was to change the status quo. If only one or two scientists said that this change was unwise, that was enough to persuade most undecided voters to vote against change. Furthermore, it took only a little bit of uncertainty about scientific knowledge to counterbalance all the professional confidence of the epidemiologists, dentists, and public health officials who had endorsed fluoridation. Advocates of fluoridation had to state their recommendations and the consequences for effectiveness and toxicity; their critics had no particular need to resolve such questions one way or another. It was to their advantage to keep the question of fluoridation in suspended uncertainty, not resolving those questions one way or another, because uncertainty demanded caution and suspended uncertainty demanded prolonged caution, which is to say inaction.

Note that the most influential antifluoridationist authors, particularly Lear, Hileman, and Smith, hesitated to say unequivocally that fluoride was toxic. Had they said so, their allegations could have been treated as testable hypotheses. Instead, they laced the fluoridation issue with equivocation.[53] Fluoride *could be* toxic; it *might be* harmful; its effects were *possibly* dangerous or *potentially* detrimental. Lear, Hileman, and Smith constantly circled back to the same platitudes: Further studies were needed. More research should be done. New evidence might arise.

Public health authorities had to concede they could not be absolutely certain that someone, somewhere, would not have a toxic reaction. As Benjamin Paul explained, this was a problem of proving a negative: "The counter-argument that bone or kidney damage is absent because it has not been detected does not completely rule out the possibility that damage may yet be discovered in the future."[54]

This phenomenon, the heavy weight of scientific uncertainty, implicitly contrasted two kinds of scientific reasoning. Experimental science—test-tube science—is meant to discover and demonstrate cause-effect relations. When it survives standards of falsifiability and replicability, it frequently yields firm conclusions. But epidemiology emerges from a different family of scientific reasoning—namely, statistical methods that generate high levels of probability at best.[55] Given that epidemiological methods deal with large populations, absolute conclusions of 100 percent certainty were, and still are, impossible to achieve.

When people demanded certainty, they got probability instead. To worried men and women who needed absolute assurances about the safety of fluoridation, the public health authorities' honest admissions of residual uncertainty must have seemed like hedging. The uncertainty people got came in miniscule doses, but those doses were more than enough to negate all the statistical confidence in favor of fluoridation.[56]

Lastly, I should mention that Brian Martin presents the flip side to my analysis. As I have described how antifluoridationists treated scientific authority and scientific knowledge, so Martin explains how advocates of fluoridation dismissed the arguments of the other side with, for example, ad hominem attacks and guilt by association. Although I disagree with his theory of power, I commend his information about "the struggle over credibility."[57]

SCIENCE AND MEANING

It would be nice, would it not, if voters neatly separated the empirical from the intangible. Put scientific knowledge here, and judge it by scientific standards: then put matters of good versus evil somewhere else, and judge them by moral standards.

Such was the hope of Bernard Mausner, Judith Mausner, Benjamin Paul, and Harvey Sapolsky. After tracing the success of the antifluoridationists to a powerful existential issue, they assembled a three-issue model of the American experience with fluoridation. That model comprised two scientific parts plus one existential part and implied that the scientific should be considered apart from the existential. This three-issue model was extremely influential. The article by Mausner and Mausner introducing the three issues appeared in *Scientific American* during the early days of the fluoridation controversies. Paul's 1961 essay, wherein the model was polished, introduced an edition of the *Journal of Social Issues* dedicated to research on the fluoridation referenda. Sapolsky's was published in *Science* just as the first wave of academic research on fluoridation waned, which gave the article an appearance of being the authoritative last word on the subject.

The scientific, however, was not so easily disentangled from the cultural. The issue of effectiveness, for example, was the strong suit of the fluoridationists because it had enormous empirical confirmation. Fluoride reduced tooth decay. But this mattered less if tooth decay was neither contagious nor fatal, as science affirmed, and if health was a personal matter, which the American creed of individual freedom affirmed. Thus, a strong scientific argument was subordinated to a stronger cultural argument.

Consider also the scientific issue of safety: was fluoride toxic? There was a large body of scientific information on this question long before the recent review by the National Research Council's ad hoc subcommittee on fluoride. But Arnold Green showed that the conflict of individual integrity versus dehumanizing bureaucracy was so highly charged with a sense of evil conspiracy and moral resistance, that when the issue of integrity versus bureaucracy intersected with the scientific question of safety, many citizens presumed that fluoride was poison.[58]

Even though this belief originated in a line of existential reasoning—freedom is precious, bureaucracies are ruthless, and so on—the cultural argument did not stand alone. Rather, it was quickened by two kinds of scientific corroboration. With the first, the pseudo-symmetry of scientific authority, a small number of people with scientific credentials had more influence among antifluoridationists than did all their colleagues who endorsed fluoridation. It mattered not whether the former were obscure, marginal, discredited, or numerically miniscule within scientific circles. It only mattered that they used their scientific credentials to extend the cultural issues into the scientific matter by saying in scientific language that fluoride was toxic.

The second kind of corroboration, the heavy weight of scientific uncertainty, made it even easier for science to affirm the moral values of the antifluoridationists. "Fluoride *might be* toxic"—these four words were far more compelling than "Fluoride is not toxic, as far as we know," provided that the former had at least a little grounding in some people's scientific credentials, some Greco-Latin scientific terminology, or some scientific citations. The institutional voices of scientific authority, such as the U.S. Public Health Service and the American Dental Association, were often powerless to persuade people otherwise.

And so by virtue of the pseudosymmetry of scientific authority and the heavy weight of uncertainty, science served the antifluoridationists, too. No doubt this distressed the advocates of fluoridation, who felt that those two features misrepresented scientific authority and distorted scientific knowledge. If at first they took it for granted that science had a certain intellectual integrity, that science was united within one combination of knowledge and values, they learned instead that science was available to be picked apart so as to support both sides in a polarized scientific controversy.

CHAPTER SIX

■ ■ ■

Plague

The early years of the AIDS/HIV epidemic provided enormous opportunities for alternative theories to coexist credibly alongside the orthodox pronouncements of established scientific and medical authorities, especially those of the U.S. government. After all, the government scientists' explanations of the epidemiology and etiology of AIDS/HIV were unavoidably tentative, hypothetical, and incomplete, even while fear of AIDS was very real. People needed to hear it said unequivocally that the AIDS virus would not kill them. If government scientists could not provide that comfort, then much of the public would turn to other voices for reassurance.

Daniel Fox describes that situation as a crisis of medical authority. Again and again throughout this century, government-sponsored science improved many millions of lives by curing infectious diseases, and even eradicating some of them, so much so, in fact, that it came to be taken for granted that American medical science could overcome any infectious disease. But by saving so many lives from afflictions that ordinarily struck people when they were young or middle-aged, this kind of success increased the number of people who reached old age. That, in turn, increased the number susceptible to chronic diseases—arthritis, Alzheimer's, and so on—for which medical science could do little. Unfortunately, many a doctor, scientist, and consumer carelessly extended their confidence about infectious diseases to expectations about chronic diseases, thereby underestimating the intractable strength of the latter.[1] After all, if medical science could cure one kind of disease, why could it not also cure another kind?

The rise of the AIDS/HIV epidemic in the early 1980s revealed the limits of medical authority for both infectious and chronic diseases.

This was an infectious disease, but it would not be cured easily or even controlled soon. It was also a chronic disease, guaranteed to produce long-term suffering for large numbers of people.[2]

If hindsight came in flavors, then hindsight about the early days of AIDS would have a bittersweet taste of tragedy entwined with innocence. As late as May 1982, many gay men in San Francisco were clinging to naive miasma theories to explain the epidemic because it would have nothing to do with homosexuality if the cause was something in the water, something in the air, something in drinks, or something mechanical in the atmospheric ionizers in bars, writes Randy Shilts.[3] Epidemiologists sought their answers in "gay lifestyle" hypotheses centered on drugs and sex, particularly poppers and promiscuity.[4] That way, AIDS would be a minor problem of personal mischief, amenable to a little tinkering in "behavior modification" within a sharply defined subculture of homosexuality. It would hardly be frightening at all and would be far less worrisome than a lethal pathogen that might reach into almost every human population.

Most of the public, however, was far from comforted. S. C. Combie notes that Americans tend to exaggerate the dangers of contagion, as if all infectious diseases are transmitted as easily as tuberculosis.[5] When AIDS was grouped with other infectious diseases, including syphilis and influenza, it mattered very little that some were more easily transmitted than others: "infectious" was taken to mean highly contagious.[6] Among the mass media, furthermore, a long-established habit of sensationalist reporting on health and illness described each new disease in the most dreadful terms.[7] Formulaic reporting on AIDS/HIV was faithful to this bad habit, emphasizing danger to heterosexuals, misinterpreting new scientific hypotheses in the most dire ways imaginable, but also recklessly predicting that miraculous cures were almost at hand.[8]

And so AIDS gave the public a reason to panic, after which government scientists were expected to quickly fix the cause of this panic. According to Dennis Altman, "The failures, to date, of medicine to find either a cure for or a means of prevention of AIDS may be more galling for Americans to accept than most people. The American belief that any problem can be solved if one throws enough money at it makes it tempting to locate blame for the continuance of the epidemic, and to harbor the suspicion that the government could end it if it wanted."[9]

American medical authorities, of course, had not been idle. Those at the Centers for Disease Control had established all the routes of HIV transmission by 1983, and their French colleagues accurately described the virus in February 1984.[10] Then between 1984 and 1987, government-sponsored science achieved a consensus of understanding about AIDS. This "Orthodox Paradigm," as I call it, embraced these categories of knowledge and belief:

1. *Etiology:* the HIV retrovirus is the pathogen that causes AIDS by destroying T4 cells, thus compromising the immune system and leaving the individual vulnerable to opportunistic infections.
2. *Epidemiology:* the HIV virus is transmitted via the exchange of bodily fluids, principally blood, semen, and vaginal fluids. The main mechanisms accounting for almost all infection have been sexual activity (*not* restricted to homosexual practices), needle-sharing intravenous drug use, blood transfusions, and perinatal transmission (mother-infant contact at birth).
3. *Prevention:* because there is no cure for AIDS, and because the transmission of HIV requires certain kinds of behavior, control of the epidemic requires education and behavior that result in blocking the exchange of HIV-infected bodily fluids. "Safer sex," especially condom use, and clean-needle activities are recommended.

Nevertheless, the U.S. government's doctors and scientists had failed the public in the sense that they had neither cured AIDS nor controlled it. On the contrary, rates of HIV infection doubled every twelve months throughout the mid-1980s. The government's main strategy for prevention was to steer public attitudes on a middle path that was neither apathy nor hysteria: be very concerned about AIDS, but do not panic. This message was too subtle for many. Some populations tended toward apathy and others toward panic, fueled by contagion fears and sensationalist media. Still others combined panic *and* apathy—that is, panic about getting AIDS through casual contact and apathy about responsible behavior, such as using condoms.

Another complication was the hostile suspicion, especially among knowledgeable AIDS activists, that government scientists responsible for ending this epidemic were morally corrupt. One of the main themes of Randy Shilts's book *And the Band Played On* is that Robert

Gallo and his associates in the National Institutes of Health were too much concerned about glory and reward and too little concerned about the suffering of people with AIDS/HIV.[11]

At any rate, the cumulative effect of these failures, suspicions, and phobias was a common feeling that government scientists were not up to the task of protecting America from AIDS. Not surprisingly, then, there arose a thriving subculture of alternative theories about AIDS/HIV. The more the government disappointed the nation in the matter of AIDS/HIV, the more attractive the various alternative theories seemed.

The alternative theories come in two families: theoretical therapies and theoretical explanations of AIDS. Such therapies include Compound Q, a Chinese potion derived from cucumber roots; DNCB (dinitrochlorobenzene), a skin medication for warts; Dextran Sulphate; and Kemron, a form of alpha interferon. Faith in these therapies was nurtured by a subculture of anecdotes, newsletters, smuggling networks, and buyers' clubs. Of the theoretical explanations, two of the most prominent have been Peter Duesberg's and Tom Curtis's.[12] According to the former, the HIV virus is benign, hence unrelated to the symptoms of AIDS, in which case the multiple symptoms have multiple independent sources, most of which reflect reckless "gay lifestyle" behavior. Curtis's theory holds that a polio vaccine cultured in monkey kidneys was infected with a simian immunodeficiency virus (SIV) and that after the vaccine was administered to humans in central Africa, the SIV mutated into HIV.

Another interesting alternative explanation, that of Lyndon LaRouche and his associates, deserves special attention for two reasons: its advocates devoted considerable effort to matters of scientific credibility, even while challenging well-established scientific authorities, and they forced the public to make a decision about their theory by converting it into a statewide referendum in California in 1986.

THE LAROUCHE THEORY OF AIDS/HIV

Lyndon LaRouche is an idiosyncratic political leader with a band of intensely devoted followers. While pursuing a career as a businessman and economist in the 1950s and 1960s, he involved himself in the activities of obscure Trotskyite political factions. During the high tide of leftist fringe politics in the late 1960s and early 1970s, he carved out a niche for himself as a visionary theorist in the antiwar movement and related groups. To his followers, his credibility as a leader is based on the firm belief that "It is not a debatable interpretation, but is a simple matter of documented fact, that Lyndon H. LaRouche, Jr. has been established as the most accurate economic forecaster in the history of economic science."[13]

Even so, LaRouche's influence on the Left was not very impressive. During the 1970s, he executed a 180-degree shift from left-wing extremism to right-wing extremism, while retaining much of his personal following and even expanding his network of publications, institutes, and political cadres. Since 1976 he has often run for president—with little notice and less accomplishment—as an ultrarightist Democrat in the presidential primaries.

The core of LaRouche's ideology is a sweeping Manichaean conspiracy theory. According to it, the heritage of Plato, Leonardo Da Vinci, Wolfgang Mozart, LaRouche, and a few other virtuous individuals is eternally threatened by a great cabal of evil that includes the London financial center, the Swiss insurance cartel, the Venetian reinsurance cartel, the Eastern Establishment, the Socialist International, the Soviet government, the U.S. government, the Anti-Defamation League, the Jesuits, and British royalty, plus generic categories of communists, liberals, Zionists, homosexuals, and drug dealers, not to mention Aristotle, Theodore Roosevelt, Margaret Mead, and Roy Cohn.[14]

The LaRouche vision of history and culture also embraces positions on several scientific topics, including the belief that virtuous sciences such as Riemannian physics, optical biophysics, and a "mitosis-defined cell-reproduction process" are threatened by diabolical countertheories, including a "hegemonic axiomatic-deductive sort of statistical biology."[15] LaRouche anchors his scientific theories in the nineteenth-century dissertation of Bernhard Riemann, in Plato's *Timmaeus*, and in a fondness for inscribing spirals on cones.[16] From these and other considerations, LaRouche concludes that Aristotle and Galileo were "hoaxster[s]" and that much of commonly accepted scientific knowledge is "absurd."[17]

At one time or another, Lyndon LaRouche has championed such scientific causes as domestic nuclear energy, fusion research, President Ronald Reagan's Strategic Defense Initiative, and a space mission to Mars. There is a predictable pattern to the behavior of LaRouche and his associates when they attach themselves to an issue, whether political, economic, or scientific. The LaRouche model of politics is as follows:

1. The issue selected is highly visible and charged with emotion.[18]
2. LaRouche and his associates research the issue very intensely, so that they have a skillful command of terms, theories, sources, and so forth.[19]
3. LaRouche presents a simplistic solution to the issue.[20] The tone of his rhetoric is authoritarian, such that there are no doubts and no qualifications in his views.
4. The solution requires a crash program for the centralized command of the economy or of national security and costs many billions of dollars.[21]
5. LaRouche and his followers allege that an evil conspiracy of diabolical forces is blocking LaRouche's solution.[22] Those who disagree with him are subjected to ad hominem attacks, particularly the accusation that they are liars and that their motivations are immoral.
6. LaRouche's personal credentials are presented in terms of his technical expertise in esoteric, even cryptic, subjects and in terms of his privileged access to leading specialists, whose identities are alluded to vaguely but not usually specified.

That last item is an important part of Lyndon LaRouche's credentials as a charismatic leader. The 1983 biography by his followers tells us that "his own work in economic science obliged Lyndon H. LaRouche to assemble and coordinate the efforts of an array of mathematicians, physicists, and other specialists, and to direct the collaborative efforts of these teams according to the specifications of his own discoveries."[23] In his 1987 autobiography, LaRouche reveals that he is "among the influential international figures of this decade."[24] Later in the book he vaguely describes his computer projections and his personal mathematical sophistication.[25] He writes, "I am in the advantageous position to know how the next great revolution in fundamental scientific knowledge will be reached. . . . I am also privileged to know concrete lines of current investigation leading in the direction of the next great sweeping revolution in science."[26]

That book is also peppered with numerous vague references to unnamed experts, authorities, and specialists with whom LaRouche consults. In addition, its photos and their captions depict him as a technical expert who is "inspect[ing]" and "examining" nuclear power facilities, the Goddard Space Center, and a high-energy accelerator. He is also shown addressing a scientific conference.

In 1973, LaRouche assembled a "Biological Holocaust Task Force," which predicted that an apocalyptic epidemic would strike in the 1980s.[27] When the discovery of AIDS seemed to fulfill this prediction, LaRouche and his associates constructed a countertheory of AIDS/HIV that digressed from the Orthodox Paradigm articulated by government scientists.[28] The main features of the LaRouche theory of AIDS/HIV are these:

1. *Etiology:* etiology according to LaRouche conforms to that of the Orthodox Paradigm—the HIV virus is the pathogen that causes AIDS.
2. *Epidemiology:* LaRouche's version of epidemiology is dramatically different from that of the Orthodox Paradigm. His version asserts that HIV, like the common cold virus, is easily spread by way of casual contact and, like malaria, by insect bites. Thus, people who are HIV-positive are extremely dangerous to the rest of the population, even if there is no intimate sexual contact, needle-sharing, blood transfusion, or perinatal transmission. Unlike the behavioral model of the Orthodox Paradigm, LaRouche's theory is a combined contagion-miasma model of the spread of AIDS.
3. *Prevention:* from that interpretation of epidemiology come these policy implications: anyone suspected of carrying the HIV virus must be tested; anyone working in schools, restaurants, or health care institutions must be tested; those who test positive must be reported by name; and they must be quarantined the way tuberculosis patients were once isolated.

This theory was developed and presented according to the usual outlines of the LaRouche political model. The topic of AIDS was already charged with emotion, and LaRouche's associates studied the scientific-medical literature carefully. As a simplistic solution, the theory offered a choice between LaRouche's "science-intensive plan[, which] will lead to total victory over AIDS," and the Orthodox Paradigm, which "will doom the human species to a miserable end."[29] The crash program LaRouche's theory recommended was described as "an emergency war plan," a "Manhattan-Project-style mobilization of basic biological research," a "battlefield epidemiological deployment," and a "Biological Strategic Defense Initiative."[30] For a sweeping program of mandatory testing, scientific research, hospital construction, and "economic renaissance," LaRouche's associates suggested an annual cost of $100 billion, and they insisted that this program be directed by LaRouche.[31]

The enemies of the LaRouche plan, including the Centers for Disease Control and the World Health Organization, were said to be "viciously lying to the world" to conceal a diabolical agenda of genocide and euthanasia.[32] Furthermore, it was repeatedly suggested that HIV had been created in a Soviet laboratory, as part of a plot to destroy the United States. This line was developed in a series of papers by John R. Seale, M.A., M.D., M.R.C.P., a London physician.[33] Seale's explanation enjoyed a semblance of being hard science by virtue of the publication of his papers in very respectable scientific journals, including *Nature* and the *Journal of the Royal Society of Medicine*. On close examination, however, these papers turned out to be letters to the editor and highly speculative opinion pieces.

THE CAMPAIGN FOR PROPOSITION 64

In 1986 LaRouche and his associates converted his theory of AIDS/ HIV into a referendum on public health policies, and they gathered enough signatures to place it on the California ballot, to be decided by popular vote, for November 1986. "Proposition 64," as it was titled (also known as the LaRouche Initiative), required that AIDS be classified as a disease that is spread easily (implying, that is, by casual contact, like the common cold, and by insect transmission, like malaria). The proposition also required mandatory testing for anyone suspected of carrying HIV and for workers in schools, hospitals, and restaurants. Finally, the initiative suggested that those who were HIV-positive should be reported by name and that they be quarantined.

To promote Proposition 64, the LaRouche organization created a lobby called Prevent AIDS Now Initiative Committee, or PANIC, and they supported it with scientific and medical testimonials from the existing Biological Holocaust Task Force. Opposing the LaRouche Initiative were the deans and faculties of four leading California schools of public health, who collectively asserted, "The LaRouche Initiative runs counter to all public health principles."[34] Also included in the opposition were leading scientists at Stanford University, notably David Korn (dean of the medical school and chair of the presidentially appointed National Cancer Advisory Board), who argued that Proposition 64 was "based on patently inaccurate scientific information."[35] Additional opponents were the surgeon general, the Red Cross, numerous other health professionals, gay organizations, labor unions, and the Democratic Party of California.[36]

The comments and behavior of LaRouche and PANIC may seem bizarre, if not downright offensive, since their advocacy of Proposition 64 digressed wildly from the Orthodox Paradigm of AIDS/HIV, along with all the conventional scientific judgment that ratified the Orthodox Paradigm. Nevertheless, the campaign in favor of the referendum ought not to be dismissed as an inexplicable outbreak of irrationality, for it was a faithful exercise in the LaRouche model of politics. The campaign employed three strategies: (1) to challenge the scientific competence of the government's science bureaucracy, (2) to argue that LaRouche had special scientific insights by virtue of his personal qualities, and (3) to claim that LaRouche's insurgent scientific experts were more competent in scientific matters than the government's experts.

STRATEGY 1: CHALLENGING THE COMPETENCE OF BUREAUCRATIC SCIENCE

When the public panics in the face of a disease, there is obviously little confidence in the government's biological and medical research institutions or in state and federal public health departments. Neither can those organizations easily reestablish confidence in a climate of panic. Thus, LaRouche and his associates launched an indirect assault on government science by amplifying fear of AIDS. They announced that AIDS was "worse than the Black Death" and "a disease more deadly to mankind than a full-scale thermonuclear war."[37] Furthermore, they described HIV-positive people as the "walking dead."[38] On the basis of their theory of casual contact, PANIC warned that a rally against the LaRouche Initiative was a public health threat because it included many gays.[39] For these and other reasons, a California judge ruled that statements submitted by PANIC were meant to create a "dread, awful aura."[40]

A more direct challenge was a series of ad hominem attacks and generic defamations directed against those who disagreed with LaRouche. Dr. Mathilda Krim, founder of the American Foundation for AIDS Research, was accused of terrorist activities in France.[41] Judge James Ford of the Sacramento County Superior Court, who had reprimanded PANIC and emended its statements, was denounced as "an intimidated and incompetent judge."[42] LaRouche referred to opponents of Proposition 64 as "the sort of Alaistair Crowley, Aldous Huxley type of counter-culture people who say . . . that they have established legitimacy for this counter-culture [of rock music, sex, and drugs]."[43]

Numerous scientists were automatically labeled liars for no other apparent reason than that they disagreed with LaRouche. The chair of the California Medical Association was said to be lying, and the Centers for Disease Control were accused of suppressing evidence of insect transmission.[44] "Those who say there is very little danger from 'casual contact' are liars. They are guilty of one of the most evil cover-ups in medical history."[45] In general, said LaRouche, most AIDS/HIV researchers and public health officials were lying.[46]

STRATEGY 2: PRESENTING THE CHARISMATIC QUALITIES OF LAROUCHE

There were two forms of the claim that LaRouche was personally gifted with extraordinary insights. In the first form, it was stated or implied that he was closely associated with some of the world's leading scientific experts and leaders, as had been stated in previous LaRouche publications. During the 1986 campaign, for example, LaRouche announced, "I have received reports from some of the world's leading figures in medical science,"and "Since I am fortunate to be influential in scientific circles internationally, I have used that influence to organize support for AIDS research."[47]

In the second form, LaRouche himself was said to be a leading expert in his own right in certain scientific fields, which, he implied, would be the most important scientific knowledge in the near future. Thus, in his interview with *New Statesman,* he suggested he was a leading expert in "non-linear spectroscopy," "optical biophysics," and "Riemannian physics."[48]

In both kinds of claims of charismatic leadership, there was a high degree of cryptic allusion. For one thing, the world leaders with whom he associated were typically nameless. For another, the kinds of scientific knowledge he was said to command had long technical names (e.g., "mitosis-defined cell-reproduction process"), but there was little explanation of either the knowledge behind the names or its relevance to mainstream scientific issues, including AIDS. This pattern of tossing out arcane scientific terminology was especially sharp in the case of the *New Statesman* interview. (The 1983 biography contains an eighty-page explanation of LaRouche's scientific theories and refers to him as a "Science-Administrator.")[49] And yet LaRouche's personal aura of cryptic credentials was the very stuff that made him different from government scientists who had conventional, rational, or explicit credentials.

STRATEGY 3: CLAIMING SCIENTIFIC COMPETENCE FOR THE INSURGENTS

One way to claim scientific competence for the supporters of Proposition 64 was to display the legitimate scientific or medical credentials of certain associates of LaRouche. The nine members of the Biological Holocaust Task Force exhibited six M.D.s, one Ph.D., and one D.P.H. among them. Its director, Warren J. Hammerman, and the President of PANIC, Khushro Ghandi, claimed no such credentials, but the task force and PANIC were otherwise well protected from charges of being uninformed amateurs.

A second tactic was to deploy the visual symbols of scientific realism. PANIC's principal piece of campaign literature, a twenty-four-page booklet titled "A Vote for Proposition 64 Could Save the Life of Someone in Your Family," presented fifteen graphs or charts in the first twelve pages.[50] These were followed by an appendix offering four polemical statements labeled "Affidavit 1," Affidavit 2," and so on. (Originally these had been submitted by LaRouche's associates in the proceedings in Judge Ford's court.) Since these statements were called "affidavits" outside the context of the courtroom, a reader could infer that they had a special credibility equivalent to courtroom testimony.

A third tactic was to borrow the credibility of the opposition, over its objections, by asserting that the opponents of Proposition 64 *secretly* agreed with the LaRouche theory of AIDS/HIV. For example:

- After Dr. James Chin (chief of the Infectious Disease Branch of the California Department of Health Services) met privately with the president of PANIC, the latter claimed that Chin *privately* agreed with him on mandatory testing and quarantine. Chin answered that he was being misrepresented by PANIC, but because the meeting had been private, he could not conclusively refute PANIC.[51]
- Dr. John Grauerholz of the Biological Holocaust Task Force cited Dr. Jean-Claude Chermann of the Pasteur Institute as a scientist who had proven that insects transmit HIV to humans; Chermann objected that there was no such evidence.[52]
- In a statement prepared for inclusion in the *Voter's Handbook* (published by the state of California as a guide to upcoming referendums), PANIC claimed that "numerous studies," including Chermann's, supported the insect-transmission theory. Judge Ford of the Superior Court, acting on a complaint by California secretary of state March Fong Eu, ruled that this claim had to be deleted because it was false and intended to mislead.[53]

A last way to claim the institutional authority of science was to employ the vocabulary of certainty and absolute truth in statements on scientific issues. LaRouche said that "there is no question" that insects transmit HIV, and that insect transmission of HIV "is thoroughly established."[54] He also asserted that "every leading medical institution in the United States and Western Europe knows that the deadly disease called AIDS is spread by 'casual contact.'"[55]

INTERPRETING PROPOSITION 64

Three months before election day November 1986, the *Los Angeles Times* reported that close to half of the public favored quarantine for people with AIDS.[56] In October of that year, less than a month before election day, *Science* revealed that most voters were still undecided about Proposition 64.[57] When California voters went to the polls in November 1986, Proposition 64 received slightly more than two million votes, or 29 percent of the total.

As a political event, the vote was a resounding defeat for the LaRouche Initiative and the scientific theory it represented. But it was also a precarious result, not to be taken for granted, as indicated by the earlier polls. Note that LaRouche and some of his colleagues were subjected to much-publicized investigations and trials in Massachusetts and Virginia for credit-card fraud and other charges in fall 1986. If these proceedings had not diverted enormous resources at the time of the California campaign, then there would have been much more money and staff available to support Proposition 64. In that case it might have received more votes.

A year after the 1986 vote, a national survey of "AIDS Knowledge and Attitudes" discovered that 41 percent of respondents "thought it was very or somewhat likely that you could get AIDS from being coughed or sneezed on by someone who had the AIDS virus."[58] Shortly after the 1986 California vote, PANIC gathered seven hundred thousand signatures to put the LaRouche Initiative on the ballot again for the primary elections of spring 1988. Then it received 32 percent of the vote (although the net total of votes was lower than in 1986 because fewer people vote in primaries than in general elections).

As a cultural event, the campaign gave great prominence to Lyndon LaRouche, his credentials, and his theory of AIDS/HIV.[59] Most notably, LaRouche and his allies had set the terms of the debate on California's policies for AIDS/HIV. Their campaign had drawn considerable state and national attention to policies for mandatory testing and involuntary quarantine. When TV talk shows sponsored for-and-against debates on Proposition 64, they suggested unintentionally that the arguments for these policies deserved as much attention as those against. Without endorsing Proposition 64, talk shows gave the LaRouche theory of AIDS/HIV a certain degree of respectability.[60] So, too, they aggravated public fear and confusion regarding AIDS. Also, the campaigns for and against the referendum had the effect of amplifying the celebrity cult of Lyndon LaRouche by depicting him as a central figure in a scientific controversy.

No doubt Proposition 64 appealed to homophobia, contagion fears, and other sentiments so that the vote of November 1986 reflected multiple layers of meaning that are impossible to separate and quantify. Nevertheless, those who initiated the referendum had presented their views as a scientific theory and had justified the proposition's public health policies as the rational conclusions of that theory. They had also based their campaign on the scientific merits of their policies, on the scientific credentials of Lyndon LaRouche and the

Biological Holocaust Task Force, and on the inadequacies of the government's science bureaucracy. The case of Proposition 64 was, at the very least, a democratic process for resolving a scientific question, even if most scientists felt that the scientific merits of the theory behind the proposition were negligible.

Among the various tactics used to promote the LaRouche Initiative, some were more conventional than others. Two particular tactics were ordinary ways of asserting that scientific authority supported the LaRouche theory of AIDS/HIV—namely, the display of the legitimate M.D.s and Ph.D.s of the members of the Biological Holocaust Task Force and the deployment of the visual symbols of scientific realism (the charts and graphs in PANIC's polemical literature on AIDS/HIV). Such references to credentials and to graphs are perfectly common in public disputes about science policy.

The other methods were most uncommon. The cryptic allusions to LaRouche's charisma as a scientific leader, the habit of borrowing the opposition's credibility over its objections, and the routine defamation of LaRouche's adversaries were certainly not the kinds of claims on scientific authority that scientists expect to encounter, even in a highly contentious public dispute.

Such tactics recall Gary Downey's observation on a "systematic ambiguity in the public identities of scientists in American culture." As an abstraction the institution of science is a powerful authority, but individual scientists representing particular positions in a public dispute have an unending burden of establishing their own personal credibility.[61] The usual way they do this is to claim the institutional moral authority of science for themselves, while trying to deny the same to their opponents. As a result, each party's claims on scientific authority must be constantly reasserted. Similarly, Michael Mulkay feels that because scientific information is open to multiple interpretations, scientists as expert witnesses do not necessarily help resolve disputes.[62]

In short, scientific authority is everything, but there is little common understanding of science, so each party's scientific credibility starts at zero at the beginning of each new dispute. This is an open invitation for each claimant to persuade the public that science bestows its blessings on that claimant's moral theory or political model.

That, I think, would have been true of any public debate on AIDS/HIV in the mid-1980s in light of the government's inability to stop AIDS. But the campaign style of LaRouche and his associates was so unusual that it temporarily rearranged the landscape of scientific authority, which was fragile enough already. First, the campaign for Proposition 64 multiplied the lines of argument by which LaRouche's followers could make their claims and subvert those of the government's science bureaucracy. Second, the campaign scrambled the opponent's credibility. Surely it was difficult enough for LaRouche's adversaries, even with all their degrees, titles, and institutional affiliations, to educate the California public about the Orthodox Paradigm of AIDS/HIV. But this was made even more difficult when they had to face ad hominem attacks, generic defamations, and PANIC's misappropriation of their own words.

The campaign for Proposition 64 is a particular moment in time and space, but it reflects some other conditions that are serious indeed. Science is believed to transcend culture and history, in which case it should be able to resolve disputes about physical reality. But relations between science and the rest of society are hardly transcendent. Rather, in the case of the campaign for Proposition 64, these relations were contingent on the deployment of the popular symbols of science, and other tactics, including some that are downright alien to the subculture of science. This outcome tells us that there are no consistent cultural rules for limiting a scientific dispute to tactics with which scientists are comfortable.

Finally, these conditions are not static. Because the cultural composition of scientific authority is susceptible to so many different tactics and strategies for asserting and inventing it, there is no common understanding of science that can be stabilized or even defined. On the contrary, this cultural problem is liable to become worse each time the democratic process rewards an aggressive, unorthodox challenge to institutional scientific authority.

CHAPTER SEVEN

■ ■ ■

Hope

What could be better than a technological solution to our energy problems that promised abundant power at miniscule cost, except a solution that did all that while *also* celebrating the simplicity of old-time technology? In the future we would have all the energy we wanted by virtue of a plain gadget, a simple electrolytic cell, that anyone could manage. No longer would we need legions of engineers, oil producers, bureaucrats, and policy makers to make our electricity hum. Instead, we could do it ourselves with batteries, beakers, and liquids from the neighborhood hardware store, like a teenage Thomas Edison. The hope for a quick fix plus the simplicity of kitchen-table technology: this was cold fusion.

But then, what could be worse than committing a major scientific blunder by ignoring all the obvious precautions of research procedures, except a blunder that *also* wounded millions by cruelly raising false hopes for a quick fix from kitchen-table technology? This, too, was cold fusion.

Most accounts of cold fusion have framed it as an internal drama within the scientific community. Its plot supposedly unfolded in four acts: (1) Stanley Pons and Martin Fleischmann skipped critical control experiments and presented their theory prematurely so as to protect lucrative patent rights; (2) by communicating via press conference while eschewing scientific journals, Pons and Fleischmann violated the due process of science; (3) that sin caused the details of cold fusion to be concealed from other scientists, temporarily frustrating their attempts to either replicate or falsify the Fleischmann-Pons hypothesis; (4) in the end the intrinsic strengths of science overcame the intransigence of Pons and Fleischmann, with the result that cold fusion was abjectly discredited. As a consequence of this line of reasoning, Pons and Fleischmann's behavior is now memorialized as "bad science," "pathological science," and "the scientific fiasco of the century."[1]

I have nothing to add to that internal account of scientists versus scientists, nor do I want to pass judgment on the scientific merits of the Pons-Fleischmann hypothesis. I wish to recall, however, that nonscientists suffered an emotional whipsaw of hope and the dashing of hope, an agony different from the professional frustrations of the scientists. The chemists and physicists involved in cold fusion wanted to know how to execute the procedures of organized skepticism, such as testing a null hypothesis by performing control experiments. The nonscientists wanted to know how hope would become tangible, which was diametrically opposed to the sentiments of the scientific skeptics.

While both kinds of parties needed reliable scientific knowledge about cold fusion, the nonscientists could hardly produce their own, so they had to be passive spectators to the drama of Pons and Fleischmann versus their scientific critics. If those critics within the scientific community were once removed from the necessary information because of Pons's and Fleischmann's style of communication, then the rest of us—nonscientists—were twice removed and twice as vulnerable to the agony created by false hope.

Let us say that the scientific community was like a family (and please be very generous to scientists in this analogy) and the nonscientists like another family. If so, then the nonscientists' experience with cold fusion was like trying to witness from a distance a family fight inside a household of foreigners. It was hard enough to follow the events from afar but doubly hard because the feuding family's gestures and language were alien to the witnesses.

So let us revisit the case of cold fusion, but this time to witness the parallel story, to see what nonscientists saw of cold fusion. Let us see the layers of dazzling promises and scientific disputes they saw, and let us see how cold fusion promised to change our lives. Let us ask how certain images of science aroused hope and how they dashed it.

THE COLD FUSION HYPOTHESIS

Nuclear energy can come from two different processes: fission and fusion. The first, the splitting of an atom's nucleus, is the source of commercial nuclear power and of simple atomic bombs. The second process involves the collision of two hydrogen nuclei so that they fuse. It is extremely difficult to achieve because the electrical charges of nuclei repel each other. Only at extraordinarily high temperatures will the nuclei fuse. It happens within the center of the sun and in hydrogen bombs, which use simple fission atomic bombs to create the heat to fuse the nuclei of hydrogen atoms. Although there are some active research programs to derive usable energy from high-temperature fusion, that goal has been elusive so far because the necessary temperatures are extremely difficult to achieve and even more difficult to maintain. But the prospect of controlled fusion power attracts many a scientist and engineer concerned about the energy that our world needs.

Because extremely high temperature is the obstacle to the production of fusion energy, it is natural to wonder whether fusion might not be achieved some other way. Could there be some other process for fusing nuclei that does not depend on conditions like those at the center of the sun? Over many decades, this question received much thought but led to no success.

Ironically, an unrealted scientific problem led to an experiment eerily similar to Pons and Fleischmann's cold fusion experiment. In 1924, long before fusion was understood, Fritz Paneth and Kurt Peters of the University of Berlin attempted to produce helium by forcing hydrogen gas into a palladium matrix. They reported that they had derived helium-4 (which is now known to be a telltale by-product of fusion). John Tandberg, a Swedish scientist, refined their method in 1927 by passing an electrical current through heavy water into a palladium rod. This raised the hope that helium could be produced inexpensively. Alas, the happy product of the Paneth-Peters-Tandberg method was merely an artifact of common laboratory contamination, and the hypothesis collapsed.[2]

Meanwhile, fusion research concentrated on methods involving ultra-hot temperatures. In about 1984 a pair of electrochemists put their minds to the question of producing fusion at low temperatures. Martin Fleischmann, fellow of the Royal Society and research professor of electrochemistry at the University of Southampton in England, and Stanley Pons, professor of chemistry at the University of Utah, reasoned that if the nuclei of deuterium, a variant of hydrogen, could be forced into a space too small for two nuclei, then they would have to fuse. The molecular structure of the metal palladium consisted of spaces fitting that requirement.

But what would make the deuterium nuclei squeeze into the palladium lattice? Pons and Fleischmann believed that electricity would do this. They built a simple electrolytic cell containing heavy water, for its deuterium, and having a cathode made of palladium. Their hypothesis was that the movement of the electrical current from anode to cathode would force the deuterium nuclei from the heavy water into the palladium lattice, thereby causing them to fuse. Since this kind of fusion would occur near room temperature, it would be "cold" compared to fusion at ultrahot temperatures. Fleischmann and Pons were apparently unaware that they were reinventing the work of Paneth, Peters, and Tandberg.

One issue remained for the Fleischmann-Pons method: how could one know that an electrical process had truly produced a nuclear event? There were two principal indicators. First, there should be a release of radiation, measured as a quantity of radioactive particles, that is, neutrons. Second, the energy produced by the cell, measured in terms of temperature, should be distinctly greater than the electrical energy used to power the cell.

Martin Fleischmann and Stanley Pons felt that their research was incomplete in spring 1989. They planned to continue working on cold fusion before publishing their results, but when they learned that physicists at Brigham Young University who were doing similar experiments—but with a different goal in mind—Pons and Fleischmann felt compelled to publish their research promptly. No doubt they desired the prestige of being the first to discover cold fusion. Another very powerful influence came from attorneys and administrators at the University of Utah who felt that the university's patent rights for cold fusion would be greatly strengthened, and Brigham Young University's rights weakened, if Pons and Fleischmann announced their results first. And so Martin Fleischmann and Stanley Pons said at a press conference that they had achieved cold fusion within an electrolytic cell by fusing deuterium nuclei inside a palladium lattice, with the result that the output of energy was at least four times greater than the input. This was on March 23, 1989.

HOPE WRAPPED IN HYPERBOLE

The news from Utah was enormously exciting on its own, for it reached right into the heart of all our worries about energy. But a story from the following day amplified that excitement by starkly contrasting old energy with new. March 24 was the day when the world learned about the *Exxon Valdez* oil spill. As NOVA put it, "Most of the time when we think about such disasters, we're reduced to despair. But perhaps this time, from the deserts of Utah, somebody was offering a real answer."[3]

Thus, the press had a story with "drama, heroes, wizardry, and the promise of unlimited energy," said Marcel LaFollette.[4] The heroes, the two cold fusion scientists, were "ordinary persons who had made extraordinary accomplishments, by being different."[5] If the usual experts on high-energy fusion were like Goliath, then Pons and Fleischmann were like David.[6] The promise they offered us was that "a single cubic foot of sea water could produce as much energy as ten tons of coal," which is to say that "the top few feet of water in the world's oceans contain enough [cold fusion] energy to supply the world for 30 million years."[7] "Man's greatest invention since fire" was cold fusion, said Wayne Owens, a U.S. representative from Utah.[8]

One more bit of rhetorical flourish arose when Chase Peterson, president of the University of Utah, went to Washington to request $25 million for a fusion research center to develop Pons' and Fleischmann's work. One of Peterson's consultants, Ira Magaziner, contrasted our national character with that of the Japanese. He explained to Congress, not very subtly, that

> as I speak to you now, it is almost midnight in Japan. At this very moment, there are large teams of Japanese scientists in university laboratories trying to verify this new fusion science. Even more significantly, dozens of engineering company laboratories are now working on commercializing it. . . . [Money for cold fusion] says that America is prepared to fight to win this time. . . . I have come here to ask you, for the sake of my children and all of America's next generation, to have America do it right this time.[9]

The most succinct observation about this festival of hyperbole came from Moshe Gai, an Israeli physicist at Yale, who said, "I think cold fusion is the epitome of the American dream. . . . It's the new world, it's a revolution overnight, getting rich overnight, and doing something against the understanding and against the consensus of what our scientific society is."[10]

Gai's insight came from a peculiar experience. He and his colleagues wanted to do a cold fusion experiment to falsify the Pons-Fleischmann hypothesis. "And the reaction we got from the public was that . . . you scientists are . . . the only obstacle in the way of development of science. It's because of you that the dream of . . . cold fusion, cheap energy, will not come true. Like if we got rid of you scientists, we will have a good society. . . . I was inundated by letters, telephone calls, people accusing me [of thwarting cold fusion]."[11]

As Moshe Gai was a sharp voice for scientific skepticism, so Norman H. Bangerter spoke clearly for the opposite feeling. Said the governor of Utah regarding an appropriation of $5 million for a cold fusion institute at the University of Utah, "Knowing nothing about it, I am highly optimistic."[12]

SIMPLICITY SUSTAINED IN A VISUAL IMAGE

When stories about science are illustrated, the illustrations usually convert abstract ideas into semiabstract representations, at best. The classic case is Einsteinian thought. Everyone knows that Einstein in a nutshell is "e $=$ mc^2," but this begs explanation of *e, m,* and *c*. One common way to represent this bit of science is to show Albert Einstein, or another individual looking similarly eccentric, scribbling "e $=$ mc^2" on a blackboard. This does nothing, of course, to explain anything about Einsteinian thought, but it humanizes the scientific idea by casting it in a familiar representation. One does not necessarily understand the formula, but one surely knows that it means Albert Einstein, if nothing else.

The Pons-Fleischmann hypothesis easily evaded that vexing problem of converting abstract thought into simple visual imagery, for the usual representation of cold fusion during late spring 1989 was the gadget itself: a clear glass vessel holding a see-through liquid, with one electrical connection going in and another coming out. Whether on television or in the print media, this extraordinarily simple image made it entirely unnecessary to write mathematical symbols or to draw multi-dimensional graphs, let alone explain them.

In science as in scripture, the virtue of perspicuity is uncommon but nevertheless precious. If that uncomplicated picture truly conveyed the idea of cold fusion (which it did, more or less), then two effects came from this representation. First, many millions of people who had heard about cold fusion *and* had seen a picture of the gadget could say, "Yes, I think I understand the basic idea, and I like it." Or perhaps, "I like the idea of cold fusion *because* I think I understand it."

This was a powerful combination, for a scientific idea to be both intellectually plain and visually simple, because it tapped right into one of the most influential streams of American thought about science: the Common Sense philosophy. Science *ought* to be plain and simple but had become arcane and complex. The average person *ought* to be able to see and grasp the kernel of a scientific idea but seldom could in the late twentieth century. So this visual image of cold fusion undid a little bit of a century and a half of science that had become too specialized, too complicated, too arcane. If the cultural heart of American life is the heritage of colonial times and the early days of the republic, then cold fusion was as patriotic as apple pie by virtue of being an exercise in the Common Sense philosophy.

Second, if nonspecialists could appreciate cold fusion just by watching the evening news on television, then surely competent scientists could appreciate it even more, and they could use their expertise to affirm that cold fusion was a great idea. By contrast, to be skeptical about cold fusion was to challenge something obvious— namely, a simple experiment with a clear vessel, a clear liquid, and two electrical connections. When hope and simplicity were fused, as it were, within one attractive visual image, it seemed that any scientist who doubted the cold fusion hypothesis must have a very black heart, indeed, as Moshe Gai's tormentors had attested.

SELECTIVE SCIENCE JOURNALISM

Within a day of the Utah press conference, scientists all over the world began the two-sided process of replicating or falsifying Pons and Fleischmann's claim. According to *Newsweek,* at least one thousand laboratories were soon testing it.[13] Newspapers, magazines, and television stations were hot on the scientists' heels, anxious for news about this story. For the first three months or so, scientists provided an extremely rich and very large volume of news in the form of partial confirmations, partial refutations, unqualified endorsements, qualified endorsements, dubious judgments, personal opinions, and so on. In short, the raw material for the story of cold fusion was fantastic.

Scientists at Stanford, Georgia Tech, Texas A&M, Los Alamos, the University of Florida, and the University of Washington reported positive results. So, too, did scientists in Brazil, Czechoslovakia, Hungary, India, Italy, and the Soviet Union. But others at Michigan, Oak Ridge, and the British Atomic Energy Authority described negative results. Furthermore, the Georgia Tech researchers retracted their results when they discovered a major problem in their measurement of neutrons.

Scientists from Cal Tech, MIT, and other schools developed a three-point critique of the various positive reports: (1) allegedly the obvious and necessary control experiments had not been done; (2) many measurements of heat, of neutrons, and of other signs of cold fusion had been sloppy; (3) cold fusion advocates misunderstood the body of well-established theory relevant to nuclear fusion. The most dramatic presentation of this critique came at the annual meeting of the American Physical Society in Baltimore at the beginning of May 1989. Nathan Lewis and Steven Koonin, both of Cal Tech, presented a withering commentary on cold fusion research, with Koonin telling his audience, "My conclusion, based on my experience and my knowledge of nuclear fusion, is that the Utah experiments are wrong, and that we're suffering from the incompetence and delusion of Pons and Fleischmann."[14] Two and a half months later, an advisory panel formed by the Department of Energy found that there was "no convincing evidence" the Pons-Fleischmann method had produced fusion.[15]

With so much information available, the media had to be somewhat selective in deciding what was newsworthy. This selectivity was not a question of censorship versus freedom of information but rather a classic problem of fitting one good story in among many other meritorious stories. Given that selectivity was inevitable, the question is whether it had a pattern. The science journal *Nature,* the *New York Times,* and a few other sources were skeptical about cold fusion from the start. *Science* and the *Chronicle of Higher Education* were agnostic for the first two months, presenting positive and negative results about equally. In general, however, popular media coverage tilted toward an uncritical faith in cold fusion, for the pattern of this coverage was to treat positive results as exciting news and negative results as stale stories.

If one wants to attribute blame for this pattern, the journalists deserve part of it, but the scientists get some, too. Among the print media, the *Wall Street Journal* was the head cheerleader.[16] It beat all other American newspapers by breaking the story the same day, March 23, as the press conference in Salt Lake City, and the paper's follow-up story the next day gave weight to its enthusiasm by adding scientific details from the press conference. When Brookhaven National Lab reported some results that seemed to confirm the very modest fusion research of Steven Jones at Brigham Young University, the *Wall Street Journal* overinterpreted them as confirmation of the much more contententious claims of Pons and Fleischmann.[17] Then as the skeptics emerged to challenge cold fusion, an editorial in the *Wall Street Journal* scolded them for having a bad attitude reflecting "the compulsive naysaying of the current national mood." After congratulating itself for being "ahead of the pack on the cold fusion story," the paper concluded that "people with serious ideas [i.e., people like Pons and Fleischmann] find ways to push them toward the future; that leaves plenty of people to stand around worrying about the present."[18]

John Huizenga summarized the writing of Jerry Bishop, who covered the story for the *Wall Street Journal,* by saying, "He quoted extensively from the leading believers in cold fusion, always hinting that they were on the threshold of the discovery of the century, while essentially ignoring the vast majority of scientists getting negative results."[19] When Bishop won a science journalism award from the American Physical Society for his reporting on cold fusion, some members of the society responded that his stories contained much more naïveté than science, after which they embarrassed Bishop by boycotting the ceremony for his award.

But even if the *Wall Street Journal* sinned worse than the others, it was not by much. Most of the popular media was only a little bit behind it in the spirit of gee-whiz, uncritical enthusiasm. *Business Week* took up the cause of being kind to cold fusion long after the issue had faded away. In three editorials during 1992, this magazine nurtured the hope that something might yet come of the Pons-Fleischmann hypothesis, even though the University of Utah had closed down its National Cold Fusion Institute more than a year before that.[20]

A second kind of blame for this selective reporting rests more with scientists than journalists. Those who confirmed the Pons-Fleischmann hypothesis, or thought they had, rushed to tell the world about it, often by way of a press conference. But their colleagues who got negative results were slower to say so. Douglas Morrison of the European Center for the Study of Nuclear Research had a theory about this difference:

> Since they find a positive result and it's already been published . . . they don't have to be critical because it's just confirming something. So they announce, with probably a whole press conference. . . . Whereas [those] who found nothing and who do good experiments, they're worried. Because to say a colleague is wrong is very dangerous. . . . So they worry and they're reluctant to publish. It takes time and they check and they check, and they say, "Well, maybe there's some secret we have to check on." So they're slow. So in the initial period, you only get the confirmation.[21]

It is hardly the fault of the journalists that some scientists considered cold fusion a fait accompli, thereby holding themselves to lower standards of proof, while their more skeptical colleagues adhered to higher standards. But priority has its own credibility. The believers seized the priority, and the doubters found that careful science carried a greater burden of proof than hasty science in the court of public opinion.

A third aspect of selective journalism was an unholy pact crafted by the cold fusion scientists but accepted by the journalists. When the Electrochemical Society made cold fusion the main topic of its annual meeting in Los Angeles, beginning on May 8, 1989, the program committee invited only positive reports of cold fusion and shunned those with negative results.[22] Similarly, the workshop on cold fusion convened by the Department of Energy in Santa Fe, also in May 1989, offered a series of press conferences in which the advocates of cold fusion could speak to the media without having to address the criticisms of the skeptics.[23] By the time of the University of Utah's First Annual Conference on Cold Fusion, held in Salt Lake City in March 1990, the media had become much more critical of the cold fusion hypothesis. Stanley Pons and Martin Fleischmann were the stars of the conference, of course, and they spoke in some sessions, but they were unavailable to answer tough questions from the media.[24] Various lesser advocates of cold fusion represented the cause at the meeting's press conferences, but the skeptics were again excluded from this kind of contact with the media.[25]

RED-HERRING SOCIOLOGY

The most entertaining aspect of the cold fusion story was its multi-layered human-interest angle, writ large. The believers and the doubters quickly sorted themselves into roughly recognizable social categories, so that journalists, consumers, and even scientists could spin juicy theories about the kinds of personalities that embraced cold fusion versus the kinds that questioned it.

The first conflict was that of physicists versus chemists. Much was made of a supposedly age-old tension in which physicists were habitually elitist, theoretically elegant, and condescending to chemists, who by contrast were both modest and practical. In the opinion of F. David Peat, the intellectual culture of physics has a well-controlled environment, a well-controlled system of experimentation, and relatively clear first principles. Chemistry, however, "is much closer to everyday life" because it addresses the "nitty-gritty face of nature . . . with all its idiosyncrasies and conplexities."[26] If so, then the problem of cold fusion intensified the animosity between disdainful physicists and resentful chemists.

Thus, *Newsweek* suggested that "the debate may look like a catfight between hidebound physicists and innovative chemists."[27] Some sociologists and historians adopted this conflict model to account, at least partially, for contrasting expert opinions on cold fusion.[28] Indeed, there was good evidence to support this simple sociological theory. At the April 1989 meeting of the American Chemical Society in Dallas, Texas (often referred to as the Woodstock of Cold Fusion), the president of that society crowed that after physicists had bungled the phenomenon of controlled nuclear fusion, "now it appears that chemists have come to the rescue."[29] When seven thousand of them attended the session on cold fusion, "many of the chemists, who broke into cheers at reports of impressive energy gains from the new process, appeared particularly to relish the notion that a freshman-level chemistry experiment may have succeeded where physicists had failed."[30] Two years later, chemist John Bockris of Texas A&M wrote that the only reason physicists had rejected the Pons-Fleischmann hypothesis was because "the chemists had undermined the fusion establishment."[31]

Actually, there was a peculiar glitch to this theory. Peat reported that at the May 1989 meeting of the American Physical Society, the theoretical physicists were very open-minded and enthusiastic about cold fusion, while the experimentalist physicists doubted it.[32] If so, this confounds the theory-versus-experiment alignment of physics versus chemistry as a reason for one field to doubt when the other believed.

A second layer of explanation connected skepticism and faith to elite institutions versus modest state universities, especially land-grant schools. Morrison noted, "If you took major laboratories and . . . the greater region of the *New York Times* [that is, Ivy League land] . . . it was all 'no, no, no.' If you took the remainder of the United States, the southern part, it was all 'yes, yes, yes.'"[33] He and others described a similar pattern in Europe: labs in Northern and Western Europe tended to be doubters, whereas those in Southern and Eastern Europe were mostly believers.[34] When many members of the Electrochemical Society seemed dubious about cold fusion at the May 1989 meeting, the president of the University of Utah complained, "It's less believed because it didn't happen in one of three or four major research centers."[35]

In the most extreme form of the institutional prejudice theory, Fritz Will of the University of Utah and John Bockris of Texas A&M charged that a "campaign of suppression" prevented scientists in some universities and U.S. government labs from pursuing the truth about cold fusion or even reporting positive results.[36] Eugene Mallove, a science writer at MIT, resigned from that school's news office in 1991 after echoing Will's and Bockris's claim that cold fusion research was being censored and further claiming that MIT had censored him when he had tried to expose the censorship.[37]

What should we make of these connections and accusations? Certainly the basic correlations were valid, even if there were exceptions here and there. Physicists typically doubted, and chemists typically believed, at least at first. The strongest voices of skepticism came from distinguished schools such as Cal Tech and MIT, whereas most defenders of cold fusion were affiliated with less prestigious schools, especially the University of Utah and Texas A&M University.

A sociological theory can be true, but it can also be irrelevant at the same time. If the issue at hand is whether cold fusion is valid, then the sociological commentary of physicists versus chemists is indeed germane. The issue, however, is how our culture subjects science to extrascientific meaning by loading those meanings into popular symbols of science. Specifically, I ask here how certain images of science substituted hope for science in the cold fusion controversy.

Remember that the idea of cold fusion, as formulated by Stanley Pons and Martin Fleischmann, was extremely clear and simple, both in the results it claimed to achieve and in the experimental methods that would produce those results. When the Pons-Fleischmann hypothesis confronted both chemists and physicists, the two kinds of scientists had different kinds of strengths and weaknesses for pursuing cold fusion. Nevertheless, electrochemists who knew a little nuclear physics and nuclear physicists who had learned a little electrochemistry should have been able to do the same experiment and interpret its results similarly. Before long, chemists would have falsified the hypothesis, against their own instincts, if it was invalid. So, too, physicists would have replicated it, if valid, even if they disliked their sibling discipline of chemistry. This much is certain, given the hypothesis as stated by Pons and Fleischmann. That is why I say that the sociology of physicists versus chemists, and of prestigious institutes versus state universities, is true and interesting but not particularly relevant. It is, at best, a good description of the initial sociology of science conditions but hardly a continuing determinant of the ongoing attempt to understand cold fusion.

What, then, is the relevance of this juicy sociology? Obviously it humanized the problem by affixing interesting personality types to the two intellectual stances, for and against, thus making science entertaining for millions who usually find science dense. Most of all, the pop sociology of cold fusion corroborated the cultural themes of hope and simplicity by depicting cold fusion as a moral battlefield wherein "little science had beaten big science [and] cleverness had prevailed over brute force."[38] But because this sociology was largely irrelevant to the process of assessing the actual scientific merits of the cold fusion hypothesis, it was a red herring. It diverted attention from that process to more entertaining matters.

A SUBCULTURE WITH A FUTURE

Faith in cold fusion is much diminished, but it has not died. On the contrary, it is nurtured by the belief that investments now will yield great returns in the future. "A small but vociferous band of believers," writes Frank Close, "still manages to gain the ear of leading financial journals."[39] The Electric Power Research Institute, sponsored by a consortium of utility companies, has spent $5 million or more to support cold fusion research at a lab in Menlo Park, California.[40] Toyota and the Japanese Ministry of Trade and Industry also support ongoing cold fusion research; a Toyota subsidiary called Technova has taken Martin Fleischmann and Stanley Pons under its wing, providing them with a lab in the south of France where they can pursue their 1989 hypothesis and other projects.[41]

In Salt Lake City, ENECO, "a company devoted solely to cold fusion technology," has purchased the licensing rights to the cold fusion patents owned by the University of Utah at a price of at least $100,000.[42] One can buy a package of chemistry equipment containing everything needed to do a cold fusion experiment—and measure the results—from Advanced Film Technology Inc., a subsidiary of Nippon Telephone and Telegraph, for only $560,000.[43]

Books by Frank Close, John Huizenga, and Gary Taubes have ripped into cold fusion's credibility, but another book, by Eugene Mallove, offers comfort that truth resides in the Pons-and-Fleischmann test tube after all.[44] F. David Peat's book, which was the first on this subject, ends on a note of optimism about cold fusion and includes a sharp sense of urgency about the economics of energy.[45] More recently, Mallove and others founded a short-lived journal, *Cold Fusion,* to sustain the cause. "Whatever the magazine may be," said *Science,* "it won't be pessimistic."[46]

In a rare case of a believer reaching a mainstream scientific audience directly, Edmund Storms's detailed defense of cold fusion research was published in *Technology Review*.[47] Ordinarily, however, the advocates are isolated from the doubters. Reports Storms, "It is now virtually impossible to publish positive results in certain journals because the editors or their chosen peer reviewers are convinced that the effect is bogus. This creates a catch-22: the journals will not accept papers until more papers published in such journals show evidence for the effect."[48]

An international conference on cold fusion still meets approximately once a year, and it draws scores of scientists from all over the world.[49] But this community has a peculiar intellectual subculture for a scientific body: "because the Cold Fusioners see themselves as a community under siege, there is little internal criticism. Experiments and theories tend to be accepted at face value, for fear of providing even more fuel for external critics, if anyone outside the group is bothering to listen. In these circumstance, crackpots flourish, making matters worse for those who believe that there is serious science going on here."[50]

Will most scientists accept cold fusion as good science someday? I cannot say. Will most *non*scientists separate the cultural theme of hope from the scientific problem of cold fusion? Not bloody likely.

I have three reasons for my pessimism. First, cold fusion was so thoroughly christened in hyperbole in spring 1989 that one can hardly think of it except as a shorthand term for something bigger: an exciting new technology that will easily solve all our energy problems. "Cold fusion" is now a synonym for "hope." How does one take apart a synonym and make it something less? Second, there are intractable problems in the common images and cultural processes that translate an abstract idea about nuclear science into a notion that nonscientists can appreciate. The simple visual image of the cold fusion gadget, the selective nature of science journalism, the superficial sociology that humanizes the faithful and the infidels: these features are more likely to short-circuit scientific understanding for nonscientists than to enhance it.

Of course, those are cultural features, and as such they can be changed. One could concoct a visual representation of cold fusion as complicated as a Rube Goldberg device by adding three or four dozen details from physical and chemical theory. One could invert the selectivity of science journalism, granting the benefit of the doubt to the doubters and subjecting the believers to the same kind of hostile inquisition that greets our politicians. One could re-create the pop sociology of cold fusion, turning the skeptics into admirable celebrities on the model of Stephen Jay Gould or Carl Sagan, while also demonizing their adversaries, especially Martin Fleischmann and Stanley Pons but also John Bockris and Eugene Mallove.

All this could be done, but it would hardly enhance scientific understanding for nonscientists. It would undo the spirit of hope that surrounds cold fusion and in its place insert a heroic story about brave souls who expose *false* hope as such. But this is simply trading one simplistic story for another.

Third, the two scientific subcultures of cold fusion and anti–cold fusion are now firmly in place, so that one can have personal preferences and cultural meanings confirmed without having to consider counterarguments. Even if the subculture of cold fusion is much more modest than that of the skeptics, who have conquered most of mainstream science, it still possesses enough cultural resources to nurture hope for those who want hope nurtured: scientific credentials, a glossy journal, an international conference each year, a siege mentality and a conspiracy theory to sustain it, an unending medley of partial confirmations, a sign of faith from financial interests. All these attributes are available to reassure the believer, both scientist and non-, that hope is true, even when voices from Cal Tech, MIT, and the American Physical Society say it is false.

CHAPTER EIGHT

■ ■ ■

Anarchy

Given that symbols of science can be polysemic, evolution is the one symbol that carries more different meanings than any other. To liberals, evolution indicates that progress is inevitable, which is good, but to conservatives it suggests that change is amoral, which is bad. Karl Marx and other communists believed that Darwinian thought anchored Marxist theory in nature, but John D. Rockefeller and other capitalists felt that it made predatory capitalism inevitable.

There is no limit to the practice of using evolution as a synonym for change, as in cosmic evolution, biological evolution, cultural evolution, and spiritual evolution. It matters not at all that these are different kinds of change driven by different kinds of causes. All are said to be evolution, in which case evolution means whatever one means by change, whether good, bad, inevitable, contingent, intentional, subconscious, natural, artificial, or anything else.

The irony of this problem is that the biologists and geologists who study the nuts and bolts of evolution, producing precise knowledge about natural selection, genetics, or fossils, are in the habit of separating their specific work from philosophical extrapolations. To these scientists, evolution is not a symbol of anything moral, existential, or metaphysical. It is only a body of knowledge about the history of life. Thus, the people who know the most about evolution tend to underestimate its symbolic power and its polysemic dangers.

Nevertheless, there are meanings worth understanding. One of the most important is a certain antievolutionist meaning of evolution, according to which evolution is a source of moral anarchy in American society. This theory, which circulates among creationists and their associates in the Religious Right, holds that a conspiracy named "secular humanism" causes the evil and immorality that permeate the modern world and that the idea of evolution is intimately connected to secular humanism. Therefore, to understand this sense of evolution, we must first understand the cultural meanings that fundamentalists invest in secular humanism, after which we can see how evolution becomes a symbol of secular humanism. Let us begin by putting these meanings into American history.

A BRIEF HISTORY OF THE IDEA OF SECULAR HUMANISM

For most of American history, an evangelical Protestant culture dominated our public life, especially the cultural climate of our public schools. Bible devotionals, the Common Sense philosophy, the ethos of proselytizing with one's personal witness, the piety of the born again: these features constituted much of the fabric of normative American values. Religious minorities—Catholics, Mormons, Amish, Jews, Jehovah's Witnesses, and others—usually conceded the mainstream culture to the Protestant style and then withdrew into unique religious subcultures wherein they could privately exercise their own faiths. Regardless of whether most people actually observed the Protestant code in their own behavior, it still dominated American public culture. It is not hard to see why many Protestants sincerely believed that America was an intrinsically Protestant nation.

By the late 1950s, however, the Protestant cultural domination was coming unglued. The principal indicator of this change was a series of developments in constitutional law as religious minorities established their rights to participate fully in public life without having Protestantism forced on them. Through the 1930s, 1940s, and 1950s, the U.S. Supreme Court used the Establishment Clause of the First Amendment to fix a new balance between non-Protestants and the old-time Protestantism by diminishing the legal status of the latter. The plaintiffs in almost all of these skirmishes were Catholics, Jehovah's Witnesses, Seventh-day Adventists, Unitarians, and other sincerely religious parties. Very few were atheists or agnostics. Regardless, some Protestants interpreted these events as an attack on American culture by well-organized enemies of religion.

The suspicion that an evil conspiracy of unbelief had caused those changes was fueled by the two great freedom of religion landmark cases of the early 1960s: *Engel* v. *Vitale* (1962) and *Abington* v. *Schempp* (1963).[1] In these the U.S. Supreme Court ruled that public schools must not force either group prayer or Bible devotionals, respectively, on their students. From the text of a third decision, the *Torcaso* case (1961), came a name for the supposed conspiracy: secular humanism. The plaintiff Torcaso, an atheist, had been denied the office of Notary Public by the state of Maryland because he would not affirm a belief in God, but the U.S. Supreme Court held that he was entitled to that office since Maryland's policy violated Article VI of the U.S. Constitution. Justice Hugo Black, in a minor footnote to his opinion, commented, "Among the religions in this country which do not teach what would generally be considered a belief in the existence of God are Buddhism, Taoism, Ethical Culture, Secular Humanism, and others."[2]

The Court did not define that last term, nor did it give secular humanism any special attention. If any status for secular humanism could be inferred from *Torcaso,* it was no more significant than, say, the status of Taoism.

Four years later, in the *Seeger* decision (1965), the Supreme Court concluded that a sincere personal belief in a supreme being constituted sufficient religious grounds for conscientious objector status for draftees. In doing so, both Justice Tom Clark, author of the majority opinion, and Justice William Douglas, writing a concurring opinion, mentioned that a professed atheist could not use the *Seeger* decision to achieve that status, for obvious reasons. Justice Douglas added a brief footnote that cited *Torcaso* as an example of an atheist's beliefs.[3]

Torcaso and *Seeger* came to be cited in fundamentalist folklore as a pair of decisions that made secular humanism an "official" American religion.[4] Apparently fundamentalists believed that if the Supreme Court *mentioned* secular humanism, then that made it official. This interpretation takes the two footnotes more seriously than the primary texts they accompany, and neither text shows any definition of the critical term. Furthermore, *Seeger* is worse than irrelevant to the issue of legitimating secular humanism since it gives special status to those who believe in God and denies the same to atheists. Nevertheless, *Torcaso* and *Seeger* are the origins of secular humanism's "official" standing, according to fundamentalist belief.

In *Abington* v. *Schempp*, the Supreme Court commented that "the State may not establish a 'religion of secularism' in the sense of affirmatively opposing or showing hostility to religion, thus 'preferring those who believe in no religion over those who do believe.'"[5] This brings us to two competing theories about the legal status of secular humanism: did the Supreme Court *establish* a religion of secular humanism in *Torcaso* and *Seeger,* or did it *dis*establish such a religion in *Abington?* In fundamentalist belief, the answer is both. The establishment theory crystallized resentment against the loss of the Protestant hegemony, while the disestablishment theory inspired legal assaults against secular knowledge. For example, in 1969 Max Rafferty, the ultraconservative superintendent of public instruction of California, produced a document that described a moral crisis in America and blamed it on secular humanism. Sex education, behaviorism, Marxism, and evolution, the document said, could be traced to secular humanism. Citing *Torcaso,* it said that "humanism is, by definition, a religion"; citing *Abington,* it concluded that the California public schools must not teach that religion.[6]

Three years later, in 1972, William Willoughby, religion editor of the *Washington Evening Star,* sued the National Science Foundation for "establishing secular humanism as the official religion of the United States" by publishing works on evolution.[7] Willoughby's suit failed both in federal district court and at the Supreme Court. In 1976, Representative John Conlan, a conservative Republican from Arizona, introduced an amendment to that year's education appropriations bill stipulating that no federal funds could be expended in support of "any aspect of the religion of secular humanism." His amendment passed in the House but died in the House-Senate conference. Also that year, the school board of Frederick County, Maryland, prohibited "any persuasion of humanism that promotes a religious or irreligious belief."[8] Two years later, in 1978, Dale Crowley of the National Bible Knowledge Association sued the Smithsonian Institution on the grounds that an evolution exhibit constituted an establishment of the religion of secular humanism. His initiative failed in federal court.[9]

A more significant event of 1978 was the appearance of a law review article by John Whitehead and John Conlan that offered a theory of the history of secular humanism and gave the term some substantive content.[10] The historical theory began with the claim that colonial American society was so intrinsically Protestant that Protestantism should still rule American life; secular humanism, however, had usurped that hegemony by employing a series of wrong-minded Supreme Court decisions, beginning in 1878 and culminating in the

Seeger case of 1965. Currently, the authors asserted, secular humanism was so deeply embedded in public life and government policy
that it occupied the status that only Protestantism deserved to own.
And yet secular humanism's very success made it an established religion in First Amendment terms. Thus, Whitehead and Conlan offered
fundamentalist leaders great comfort by predicting that the First
Amendment could wreck their enemy as surely as it had wrecked public school prayer.[11]

Furthermore, the authors fixed a serious problem in the argument
against secular humanism by doing something the Supreme Court had
never done: define the phrase. After studying a pair of documents by
the American Humanist Association called *Humanist Manifesto I* and
II, Whitehead and Conlan stated that "secular humanism is a religion
whose doctrine worships Man as the source of all knowledge and truth,
whereas theism worships God as the source of all wisdom and truth,"
and "along with the evolutionary theory, the centrality and autonomy
of Man are the prominent features of secular humanism."[12] From the
comment on autonomy, they equated Adolf Hitler and Joseph Stalin
with humanism, and elsewhere they labeled secular humanists "those
who believe in no morals."[13] Thus, after seventeen years of citing one
sparse footnote from *Torcaso* and a second, even sparser one from
Seeger, fundamentalist Christians finally had something about secular
humanism they could describe in detail.

Even at that point, hostility to secular humanism was an obscure
legal theory. But in 1980 a book titled *The Battle for the Mind,* by Reverend Tim LaHaye, of El Cajon, California, galvanized fundamentalist
fears of humanism by rendering a popular version of the Whitehead
and Conlan thesis. LaHaye followed the Whitehead and Conlan definition of humanism, which emphasized autonomy, and he illustrated
the evils of humanism by referring frequently to pornography, homosexuality, drug addiction, abortion, and the giving away of the Panama
Canal to communists. The cumulative product was a lowbrow Mani-
chaeanism. LaHaye attested that "most of the evils in the world today can be traced to humanism" and that "crime and violence in our
streets, promiscuity, divorce, shattered dreams, and broken hearts can
be laid right at the door of secular humanism."[14] (In LaHaye's book,
"humanism" is shorthand for "secular humanism," as if all humanism is equivalent to secular humanism.) Finally, LaHaye elevated two
documents, the *Humanist Manifesto I* and *II,* to the status of sacred

scripture for humanists: "What the Bible is to Christians, the Humanist Manifesto is to humanists."[15]

The impact of LaHaye's book was startling. "In 1979 many fundamentalists had not even heard of secular humanism," write Jeffrey Hadden and Charles Swann. "It was not mentioned in sermons and writings. But by the end of 1980 nearly all had adopted it as their enemy."[16] Reverend Lamarr Mooneyham, the Moral Majority leader of North Carolina, said, "I wasn't aware of the growing influence of secular humanism before the early 1980s. But as I began to address issues facing Moral Majority chapters, at the root of every opposition was an active or passive humanist."[17] According to *Newsweek*, 350,000 copies of *The Battle for the Mind* had been sold by mid-1981.[18]

THE CULTURAL MEANINGS OF SECULAR HUMANISM

In general, conservative Christians have adopted two styles for expressing the meaning of secular humanism. I call these the "negation of personal beliefs" and the "autonomy theory," respectively. Consider these four examples of secular humanism as a negation of one's personal beliefs:

- The *Bible-Science Newsletter* lists nine components of humanism: naturalism, evolution, faith in humanity, faith in reason and science, relativism, situational ethics, antiauthoritarianism, civil liberties, and globalism.[19]
- A tract titled "Humanism: America's Greatest Enemy" gives these features of humanism: "OK to lie, OK to kill, OK to steal, OK to have pre-marital sex, OK to cheat," plus transcendental meditation, yoga, witchcraft, masturbation, children playing the roles of homosexuals and unwed parents, survival games, communism, atheism, evolution, and amorality.[20]
- A letter to the *Charlotte Observer* states that "abortion, pornography, evolution, sex and values education, socialism, communism, and bureaucratic government" are all part of secular humanism.[21]
- A pamphlet titled "Is Humanism Molesting Your Child?" says that humanism includes the denial of these beliefs: deity of God, inspiration of the Bible, divinity of Jesus Christ, existence of the

soul, life after death, biblical account of creation, and absolute standards of right and wrong. Furthermore, the pamphlet alleges that humanism embraces sexual freedom "regardless of age," plus incest, removal of male-female distinctions, control of the environment, "removal of American patriotism," disarmament, and, finally, "one-world socialist government."[22]

Notice how this style of expression attributes cultural meaning to secular humanism. Its authors list their own most precious spiritual values, and then from these templates define secular humanism as the exact opposite of their credo. Likewise, they give us very honest views of their most troubling fears and then add these to their lists of secular humanism's particular attributes, value for value and fear for fear. These definitions reveal much about their author's cares and fears, but they assign nothing to secular humanism except the exact opposite of all that the authors believe in.

A comparison of the four examples reveals another important fact. There is some overlap of particulars among the four, but many items are unique to one example or another. The first includes civil liberties but not masturbation, the second mentions masturbation but not bureaucratic government, the third has bureaucratic government but not euthanasia, and so on. Each author customizes his or her own portrait of secular humanism. The cumulative effect is multiple solipsism. Secular humanism means something different to each enemy of secular humanism.

The second style of defining secular humanism, the autonomy theory, holds that atheism constitutes a vacuum of ethical values, which is then filled by an attitude of extreme human autonomy: each person must be his or her own supreme being since there is no higher being. Autonomy then leads to anarchy because each individual will live in a world of moral relativism and situation ethics, not recognizing any common standard of morality. Thus, secular humanism is thought to be a slippery slope from atheism to autonomy to anarchy.

Recall that LaHaye's book and the article by Whitehead and Conlan emphasized autonomy in their definitions. The following passage from a creationist newsletter echoes those views: "When man substitutes his own knowledge and wisdom for the Creator's and allows every man to believe he is a law unto himself, there is no need to recognize the conscientious 'absolutes' imposed on him by government. But where does this thinking lead? Can we as a nation survive if we believe in the absolute authority of men and deny the law of God? Can we allow the standard to be the lowest common level to which man can sink?"[23] Hostility to human autonomy also arises in the comments of creationism's grassroots activists in North Carolina, many of whom I interviewed in the early 1980s. They asserted that secular humanism constitutes "a worship of man alone," "man as the Supreme Being," "a king-size ego trip," "elevation of man to the God level," "the captain of his destiny, apart from any deity," "man himself determines what is right and what is wrong," "a man-centered religion," "man is the measure of all things," "man is not responsible to a superior being."

These grassroots expressions indicate how completely the Whitehead-Conlan-LaHaye autonomy definition has been accepted. By contrast, none of my interviewees in North Carolina described secular humanism according to the negation-of-beliefs approach, thus suggesting that it is a literary device reserved for the Religious Right's tracts, pamphlets, and letters to newspapers.

An important relation between the two styles is that the autonomy theory is distinctly more focused than the negation-of-personal-beliefs approach, for it offers debatable hypotheses about philosophical linkages and social causation. But the idiosyncratic expressions of discontent from the negation-of-beliefs style lack such clarity. For example, the autonomy theory states a hypothetical relation between atheism and autonomy such that atheism is the ultimate cause of anarchy, whereas the proximate cause is autonomy. By contrast, the other approach carelessly lumps together atheism and autonomy, along with many other items.

Either way, the term "secular humanism" gives a name to the deep moral outrage felt by fundamentalist Christians. The phrase is invariably followed by a complaint about spiritual depravity in this land.

THE CULTURAL REALITIES OF
SECULAR HUMANISM

The views of Conlan, Whitehead, and LaHaye constitute a conspiracy theory. They presume that there is a distinct ideology named secular humanism, that it has agents (the secular humanists), and that they control much of American culture, especially U.S. Supreme Court decisions and public school curriculums. This theory is much more dire than the observation that American culture is becoming more secular as the Protestant hegemony is gradually retired (which indeed is happening). In fact, the conspiracy theory interprets all instances of secularization as having been spawned by a single, highly organized force.

Indeed, there is a certain modest reality to secular humanism. There is an American Humanist Association, and its *Humanist Manifesto I,* from 1933, is an explicitly antitheistic statement.[24] Its next proclamation, the *Humanist Manifesto II,* from 1973, is peppered with religion-baiting hostility, and it makes claims about human autonomy, just as LaHaye charges.[25] The humanism described in Paul Kurtz's definitive essay is truly a combination of atheism and individual freedom. To Kurtz, the history of humanism is the history of hostility to religion, with religion defined in terms of ignorance and superstition. "Basically," says Kurtz, "secular humanists are atheists, agnostics, or skeptics," and "the salient virtue [of humanism] is autonomy."[26] With those words, plus the two manifestos, the American Humanist Association delivers to LaHaye more than enough material to build the argument that secular humanism can be reduced to atheism and autonomy.

Even so, these facts deserve a sense of proportion. The seven national humanist organizations have a gross total of 12,092 members (although the net total is smaller if some groups have overlapping memberships).[27] Compare these numbers with LaHaye's figure of 275,000 humanists, which he established by citing an off-the-cuff estimate from the *New York Times,* to which he gratuitously added 10 percent, thereby giving the rough estimate the appearance of a precise quantity.[28] In reality, the *Humanist Manifesto I* and *II* are obscure documents, better known to fundamentalists than to their enemies. There are barely enough Secular Humanists to populate a modest fringe movement, let alone control the moral climate of American culture. If the miniscule numbers of the American Humanist Association are seen in proportion, then it is impossible to accept either the claim that secular humanism governs all that is bad in Western civilization or the counterclaim that it produces all that is good.

It is common for fundamentalists to believe that humanism and secularism can be folded into each other, yet a rich tradition of Christian humanism coexists with the secular form. Quattrocento Italian Renaissance humanism was very much compatible with Christian belief.[29] One of its offspring was Christian humanism, best represented by the writings of Desiderius Erasmus. Its scriptural referents are the life of Jesus and Psalm 8:4–5: "What is man, that Thou art mindful of him? And the son of man, that Thou visitist him? For Thou has made him a little lower than the angels, and has crowned him with glory and honour." Spanning five centuries, the tradition of Christian humanism embraces the ministries of Martin Luther and Martin Luther King, as well as those of Albert Schweitzer, Angelo Roncalli, Jacques Maritain, and Mother Teresa.[30]

Likewise, secularism cannot be reduced to humanism. Stalinism and Nazi fascism were secular enemies of the Judaeo-Christian religion, but no humanist would claim that either was humanistic. The "New Age" movement is a secular alternative to Judaeo-Christian spirituality, but it is hardly humanistic.[31] And so if some humanism is secular, but much else is not, and if some secularism is humanistic, while much else is not, then the fundamentalist conspiracy theory of secular humanism is a profound distortion of humanism and is grounded in a great exaggeration of the modest reality of the American Humanist Association.

IRRESPONSIBLE MOLECULES: EVOLUTION MEETS SECULAR HUMANISM

If evolution is to be tied to immorality, it must be incorporated into secular humanism. This is done in both styles of characterizing secular humanism. In the negation-of-personal-beliefs approach, belief in evolution is often listed as one of the many items that collectively constitute secular humanism. The first three examples of that approach that I gave included evolution. But others omit it while emphasizing sexual issues, or communism or New Age thought or whatever in their own inventories of secular humanism.

A more serious matter is evolution's purported relation to the autonomy theory. Evolution is accused of promoting the slippery slope from autonomy to anarchy by implying that randomness in nature justifies anarchy in society. If so, then people who believe in evolution will think anarchy is good and natural. Thus, evolution is charged with being the natural history of anarchy.

Note that the task of fitting evolution into that theory requires one to represent it as a celebration of randomness: evolution is described in terms of its random features, especially mutation. In 1972 creationists in California accused evolutionists of teaching that "the universe, life, and men are simply 'accidents' that occurred by fortuitous chance without cause, purpose, or reason."[32] Also in that year, Henry Morris of the Institute for Creation Research (ICR) wrote, "The very essence of evolution, in fact, is random mutation, not scientific progress."[33] Later, the ICR stated, "Christ offers purpose and hope for eternity; evolution proffers randomness and uncertainty forever."[34] In the 1978 lawsuit against the Smithsonian, Dale Crowley described evolution as "the assumption that man and all life on earth is the consequence of a series of accidents of molecular combination in the dateless past."[35] Morris, in his history of creationism, alleges that evolution "necessarily means endless ages of random changes which, in the process, leave untold waste and pain and death in their wake."[36]

So the problem with evolutionary thought is that, if people believe molecules behave irresponsibly in nature, then the same people will believe it is all right for individuals to behave irresponsibly in society. The most succinct denunciation of this natural history of anarchy comes from R. L. Wysong, who writes, "If life came into existence through purely natural, materialistic, chance processes, then, as a consequence, we must conclude life is without moral direction and intelligent purpose. . . . Atoms have no morals, thus, if they are our progenitors, man is amoral."[37] The same complaint resonates in the comments of some of the creationists in North Carolina:

- "If one accepts the evolutionist point of view . . . he's just a random product of molecular collisions. So man is answerable to himself, which I think is dangerous. He then has the freedom to set his own moral standards."
- "The evolution model says life arose from nothing, by pure random chance. . . . This theory of origins is leading to the view that you're not responsible to a higher authority, that man is only responsible to himself. . . . Life is a totally random event. Nothing really happens."
- "Secular humanism is the idea that man himself determines what is right and what is wrong, that he doesn't have to answer to any higher being. . . . An evolutionist who believes that

things came about by chance would also say, we are not answerable to any higher being."

From these statements a simple parallelism can be constructed:
evolution is to secular humanism as random molecules are to irresponsible individuals. But this formulation eliminates classic Darwinian
thought from evolution. It draws attention to mutation and other random processes of evolution, but it deletes evolution's deterministic features, such as adaptation and differential reproductive success, which
together constitute the process of natural selection. In fact, conventional evolutionary thought considers evolution to be an interaction
between random and deterministic processes. Ernst Mayr puts it this
way;

> As for the objection to the presumed random aspect of natural
> selection, it is not hard to deal with. The process is not at all a
> matter of pure chance. Although variations arise through random
> processes, those variations are sorted by the second step in the
> process: selection by survival, which is very much an anti-chance
> factor. . . . Selectionist evolution, in other words, is neither a chance
> phenomenon nor a deterministic phenomenon, but a two-step tan-
> dem process combining the advantages of both.[38]

Some opponents of creationism have objected to this habit of ed-
iting out natural selection. Norman Newell complains that, contrary
to creationist representations, "most biologists now recognize natural
selection as the directive force in evolution. No modern evolutionist
believes that evolution is the result of a long series of random accidents."[39] William Pollitzer, reflecting on his 1974 debate with Henry
Morris, recalls, "My opponent [Morris] suggested that evolution must
be equated with chance. Yet I see nothing in evolution that denies the
laws of cause and effect operating in an orderly universe. . . . It is natural selection in its interplay with the changing environment that en-
sures direction, in contrast to the disorder implied by the word
'chance.'"[40]

This representation has become fixed into creationist thought because that thought stems from fundamentalism's critique of immorality in American society, as organized according to the cultural
meaning of secular humanism. It must conform to the ideological

structure of that critique, in particular to uphold autonomy theory's accusations about anarchy, which means that creationism must amplify randomness and mute Darwinian determinism in its representations of evolution.

Lastly, there is one more means of connecting evolution to immorality. It alleges that evolution is *directly* responsible for immorality, without reference to secular humanism. Earlier in this century, that was the way William Jennings Bryan denounced evolution when for example, in 1922 he charged that evolutionists "weaken faith in God, discourage prayer, raise doubt as to a future life, reduce Christ to the stature of a man, and make the Bible a 'scrap of paper.'"[41] In the more contemporary version of this accusation, Judge Braswell Dean of the Georgia Court of Appeals says, "This monkey mythology of Darwin is the cause of permissiveness, promiscuity, pills, prophylactics, perversions, pregnancies, abortions, pornography, pollution, poisoning, and proliferation of crimes of all types."[42]

The most prolific and most vehement source of this view is Morris of the ICR, who asserts that "the deception of evolution" was responsible for Satan's rebellion against God, Eve's deception of Adam, and Satan's deception of the world."[43] Morris also suggests that Satan invented evolution at the Tower of Babel.[44] Morris writes, "The foundation of false teaching in every discipline of study, and therefore of ungodly practice in all areas of life, was evolutionism."[45] He presents specific examples as follows: "If man is an evolved animal, then the morals of the barnyard and the jungle are more 'natural,' and therefore more 'healthy,' than the artificially-imposed restrictions of premarital chastity and marital fidelity. Instead of monogamy, why not promiscuity and polygamy? . . . Self-preservation is the first law of nature; only the fittest will survive. . . . Eat, drink, and be merry, for life is short and that's the end. So says evolution!"[46]

Morris traces pagan religions, humanism, and the "New Age Movement" to evolution, and also holds it responsible for "most of the spiritual and moral problems that have arisen to hinder the gospel."[47] Elsewhere, Thomas McIver and Lester Harrison give additional examples of the accusation that evolution is directly responsible for immorality.[48] As blistering as these diatribes are, they fail to specify how evolution could have caused so much immorality. In this regard they resemble the negation of personal beliefs.

Although it is impossible to quantify the authority of each of the three approaches (negation of beliefs, autonomy theory, and theory of direct responsibility), the autonomy theory is probably the most influential condemnation of evolution, for it offers a relatively clear plan by which evolution is said to be tied to the grand scheme of immorality named secular humanism. The other two approaches draw much attention by virtue of their lurid and sweeping allegations, but they fail to answer the central ideological question that excites modern creationism: how is evolution connected to immorality?

A CREATIONIST SOCIOLOGY OF EVOLUTIONISTS

If evolution generates immorality, whether directly or indirectly, then those who defend evolution are agents of immorality, whether intentionally or not. That idea establishes a series of denunciations of the moral character of evolutionists. First and most frequent is the charge that evolutionists are "pompous and arrogant, just the kind of people that the First Amendment was written to protect us against," and that they display "an academic arrogance frequently typical of the nation's scientific-educational establishment."[49]

Second, evolutionists are said to be categorically intolerant. The *Bible-Science Newsletter* tells its readers that "fools despise wisdom and instruction. This is true of evolutionists who refuse to consider evidence which disagrees with their preconceived ideas of age."[50] The Institute for Creation Research proposes that biology teachers can be expected to grant scientific credibility to creationism "unless absolutely blind, or dulled by prejudice."[51] Elsewhere the ICR cites a survey of network television executives, who, it reports, are very tolerant of adultery, homosexuality, abortion, and liberalism, from which it infers that, "although the creation/evolution question was not specifically addressed in the survey, it is obvious that such a group of people would be heavily biased in favor of evolution."[52]

Third, evolutionists are thought to be systematically deceitful. It is a regular feature of creationism to allege that the Java Man and Peking Man fossils are as fraudulent as Piltdown Man. The *Creation Science Prayer News* warns that "evolution traps" have "been set by atheistic humanists all over our country . . . [so that] the tourist . . . [inhales] large doses of evolutionary indoctrination."[53] Among the evolution traps it identifies are the Grand Canyon and zoos and aquariums in general.

All the usual impeachments of evolutionists' moral character are captured concisely by Dr. Duane Gish of the ICR in his closing remarks at an October 1981 debate at Liberty Baptist College. In two short paragraphs of text, Gish accuses evolutionists of being dogmatic, intolerant, deceitful, arrogant, elitist, afraid of creationism's truths, afraid of majority sentiment, and accustomed to indoctrinating their students.[54] These judgments are especially vivid in the fundamentalist comic-book tracts of Jack Chick, a California publisher. In *Primal Man?*, by Chick, a Christian anthropologist confronts a crew making an "evolution film." The director, Dexter, is shown to be bearded, vain, and effeminate, dressed in a purple jumpsuit with a saffron scarf. His producer acknowledges that evolution is wrong but decides to continue making his films, "even though it's brainwashing these kids. . . . Many will lose their souls because of these films."[55]

Another of Chick's comic-book tracts, *Big Daddy?*, depicts a professor of evolution as fat, bearded, and balding. He becomes hysterical when a student mentions the Bible. The other students, all of whom are evolutionists, include these figures: a black man with an Afro, dark glasses, and beads; a hippie woman with a fringed vest and long hair; a man with a peace medallion; an angry long-haired man making a clenched-fist sign; and another making a V-sign for peace. Thus, in the first two panels the artist has packed in six right-wing caricatures of leftists while associating them with evolution.[56]

Occasionally real people are denounced by name (most often Stephen Jay Gould, Carl Sagan, Paul Kurtz, and the late Isaac Asimov), but the more common pattern is to deride evolutionists and humanists in terms so sweeping and so general that all of one's enemies are interchangeable. Evolutionists are categorically arrogant, or all humanists are equally depraved. The creationist commentary on evolution and humanism is a Manichaean ideology in which two sets of moral abstractions struggle against each other to control American culture: autonomy versus piety, immorality versus biblical belief, arrogance versus humility, and deceit versus perspicuity. In other words, spiritual character and abstract virtues are thought to determine the collective destinies of humanism, evolution, creationism, and fundamentalist Christianity.

Creationist feeling about evolution, then, is much more than a narrow doctrine extrapolated from a handful of biblical verses. In fact, it represents a broad cultural discontent featuring fear of anarchy, revulsion for abortion, disdain for promiscuity, and concern about end-less other issues, with evolution integrated into those fears. Regard-less of whether one agrees or disagrees with creationist moral theories about secular humanism, this is a rich and complicated cultural un-derstanding of American culture that gives considerable existential depth to conservative Christian understandings of reality. Evolution then becomes one of the symbols of that moral theory.

Although my diagnosis of creationist feelings about evolution may seem harsh, I do not want to imply that no one has a right to raise the issue of relations between evolutionary thought and human be-havior. Certainly Social Darwinism, Karl Marx's use of Darwinism, and other philosophical uses should remind us that this idea is not going to be restricted to Galápagos finches and English pepper moths. It is inevitable that some people will make evolution a symbol of moral, existential, and metaphysical meanings, regardless of whether the con-nection is logical and regardless of whether we like it.

That is bad enough. There is no point in making the situation worse, but some still find a way to do so. During the Darwin Centen-nial of 1959, Julian Huxley predicted a new science of human possi-bilities grounded in evolution, and he announced a new theology based on evolutionary values. At one level these utterances can be seen as the harmless metaphysics of a fellow who got carried away by the spirit of the centennial, but at another level it should be realized that some people take this stuff seriously. That, in turn, gives Tim LaHaye and his followers a license to take it seriously, too, but in a very dif-ferent light.

It is one thing to describe evolution as the natural history of life on earth. But when Julian Huxley and others stretch the authority of evolutionary thought by representing it as a *moral* history of nature and humanity, then they are packing the idea of evolution with pro-found cultural meaning, in which case they bear the same burden of credibility as the creationists, the fundamentalist television preachers, and all the others whose moral theories about American culture com-pete for our support.

CHAPTER NINE

■ ■ ■

Evil

If I implicitly measured cultural meanings against scientific knowledge in the previous four chapters, there is no such danger in this one. Here the referent is not scientific knowledge per se but rather scien*tists*. We have some cultural meanings as before; and again those meanings are conveyed by an image of science conjured from the mischievous deployment of symbols. But in this case the symbols are the mad scientists of fiction and film.

FEAR OF SCIENCE

According to the cultural values of the Enlightenment, human thought and the behavior that followed from it should be rational, as opposed to emotional, mysterious, or superstitious. It should also be secular, that is, unchained from supernatural considerations. If thought and behavior were truly rational and secular, then progress could be expected: the human condition would improve. And, the ultimate fruit of the union of these values would be science—that is, a systematic study of nature driven by rationalism plus secularism and representing progress.

Even if most European intellectuals of the seventeenth and eighteenth centuries embraced Enlightenment culture, many other people were troubled by this cluster of values. They felt that emotion was a good human quality and that it should not be suppressed by cold clinical rationalism. Religious faith, particularly conventional Judaeo-Christian morality, was worth honoring. Even if it included superstition or mystery, it should not be displaced by a secular spirit. Tradition was comforting, in which case progress was threatening. If science was the apex of the Enlightenment culture, then fear of science was the core of the anti-Enlightenment culture.

This latter culture assumed slightly different forms in different places. One was German Romanticism, a celebration of mystery and emotion. The French form, known as *sensibilité,* emphasized emotion and rustic simplicity. The English contribution was Gothic literature, including both Gothic romance, which depicted true love in terms of emotional excess, and Gothic horror, which served up a combination of emotion, tradition, mystery, and superstition.

From Gothic horror came the subgenre of mad scientist stories, beginning with Mary Shelley's *Frankenstein* in 1818. As exercises in Gothic horror, these stories mined the raw material of anti-Enlightenment anxieties and then shaped them into moral narratives that purported to explain where evil in the guise of science came from and how to repel it. These stories argued that rationalist science was dangerous to one's spiritual well-being because it was too clinical, too abstract, and that the scientists who controlled the mysteries of modern secular knowledge were unaccountable to conventional standards of morality. Gothic horror stories described which kinds of depraved people used science for amoral purposes and what became of them. Also, they cautioned readers to contain secular science within the firm ethical guidelines of traditional Judaeo-Christian values.

SYMBOLS OF SCIENTIFIC EVIL

But which idioms of science symbolize the evil of science? Let us say that hypothetically three kinds of idioms could be used to represent science: (1) the physical paraphernalia of science, (2) scientific knowledge, and (3) the people who are scientists. The physical equipment is a usual element of mad scientist stories, for the title characters often need laboratories in which to perform their diabolical deeds. The role of their equipment, however, is peculiar. To appreciate this point, we must first recognize a notable difference between Gothic horror and science fiction. The latter depicts the instruments of laboratories and spaceships with exquisite detail, showing exactly how they look and how they work. Witness the way every rivet and cathode are visually caressed in television or movie series such as *Star Trek* and *Star Wars* or in the novels of Tom Clancy. The reason science fiction celebrates technology this way is because it assumes that technology is equivalent to progress and intelligence, regardless of the moral strengths or weaknesses of the good guys and bad guys who employ it. Consequently, says Susan Sontag, a science fiction story earns much of its credibility from the visual fidelity of its scientific equipment and the role of that equipment in the story.[1]

By contrast, mad scientist stories, as exercises in antirationalism, must challenge the belief that just because this stuff is scientific, it must be valuable. Yet they cannot claim that the equipment itself is evil, for antirationalism, especially Gothic horror, locates evil in the human heart. If scientific equipment is neither inherently good nor inherently evil, then it must be insignificant to both morality and narrative. How, then, should it be represented? By default this equipment comes to be depicted ambiguously, illogically, and mysteriously. Consider the experiments, the labs, the drugs, and the rays of the mad scientists. The physical artifacts of their science are presented as the miscellaneous material junk of alchemists, illogically connected and barely justified.

Consider the ambiguity of the creation scene in Mary Shelley's *Frankenstein* or the equally mysterious processes of creation in these films: *The Golem, Metropolis, Frankenstein,* and *The Bride of Frankenstein.* So, too, in Robert Louis Stevenson's *Jekyll and Hyde,* the pharmacology of Dr. Jekyll has barely any physical details but many ambiguous references to a mysterious salt. Yet this irrational way of representing the paraphernalia of science has a very important effect. It empties the rationalism out of the tangible evidence of science so that the physical paraphernalia is included in the view that all reality is ambiguous, illogical, and mysterious. In this way antirationalism tames rationalist science.

Next there is scientific knowledge. If science can be represented in terms of knowledge and that knowledge is shown to be evil, then the case is made. As Dr. Janos Rukh learns in *The Invisible Ray,* "There are some things man is not meant to know." Yet it is difficult to represent abstract knowledge in tangible terms. Rotwang (from *Metropolis*), Caligari, and others possess knowledge in the form of dusty old volumes with worn pages, but the books themselves are not nearly as frightening as the ways their knowledge affects people. To depict knowledge in terms of its effects instead of its intellectual substance, two strategies are at hand. In one strategy we learn that scientific knowledge is inherently evil because of the evidence that it corrupts people. In this category are all the mad scientist stories in which young people are innocent until exposed to scientific knowledge. According to the second strategy, if the person who uses or produces knowledge is depraved, then so is that knowledge. Scientists, then, are either those who have been corrupted by knowledge (Victor Frankenstein) or those who use it to corrupt others (the psychiatrist who torments the teenager in *I Was A Teenage Werewolf*).

In either way of saying that knowledge is evil, it remains abstract until manifested in personalities. Ultimately, the evil of science is depicted and condemned principally in terms of the character of people who are scientists. Susan Sontag remarks, "When the fear of science is paramount . . . the evil has no attribution beyond that of the perverse will of an individual scientist."[2] That the intentions of scientists are evil, that they feel no remorse for their misdeeds, that they ought to know better than to commit their diabolical deeds—these features of personal morality are combined to create the personalities of the mad scientists who then personify the evil of science.

To allege that psychiatry and psychoanalysis are dangerous, there is the real-life Dr. Franz Mesmer, but there are also Edgar Allen Poe's "The System of Dr. Tarr and Professor Feather," Fritz Lang's Dr. Mabuse films, *The Manchurian Candidate,* and the granddaddy of mad scientist films, *The Cabinet of Dr. Caligari*. To denounce the destructive power of technology, there are statistics of death and despoliation from Chernobyl and Hiroshima, but there are also *Dr. Strangelove* and Ian Fleming's *Dr. No*. To show the mischief made possible by modern medicine, we have the litany of Dr. Frankenstein, Dr. Moreau, Dr. Jekyll, and numerous other irresponsible physicians. In the words of Robert Brustein, mad scientist movies "suggest that the academic scientist, in exploring new areas, has laid the human race open to devastation either by human or interplanetary enemies—the doctor's madness, then, is merely a suitable way of expressing a conviction that the scientist's idle curiosity has shaken itself loose from prudence or principle."[3] And so the general moral strategy of the mad scientist stories is to shout, "Beware of science!" by describing an evil embodied in a scientist.

CONSTRUCTING THE SYMBOLS OF SCIENTIFIC EVIL

To trace changes in the moral character of mad scientists, it is necessary to specify some features of personality that represent morality. One can say that a fictional mad scientist is becoming more moral, or less, if he enhances his good features, or diminishes them. These three features give a good shorthand of moral character:

> *Intention.* Anglo-American law and Judaeo-Christian morality both recognize that intention is a major consideration in the judging of crime and sin. Some mad scientists are motivated by vengeance or pride (Dr. Moreau, Dr. No, Dr. Caligari, and Dr. Phibes, to name but four), whereas Dr. Jekyll and Dr. Delambre (the title character of *The Fly*) start from altruistic motives.
>
> *Remorse, reflection, and responsibility.* Some mad scientists regret having inflicted violence on the world and are troubled by what they have done. They accept responsibility for their deeds by attempting to reverse or mitigate the results. Others are, let us say, less admirable.
>
> *Level of maturity (naïveté versus experience).* Some of these characters are old enough and experienced enough to know better than to unleash evil. Others, including the kind we call a sorcerer's apprentice, do so because of youthful folly. If the latter ones change, then they become more mature, as does Victor Frankenstein in Mary Shelley's novel.

These features are common moral standards. Because they are so common and so real, they make the fictional mad scientists more believable when those scientists' personalities are constructed from some combination of the three moral standards. We can say that every fictional mad scientist possesses at least one evil aspect from among those standards. Some scientists, however, have benevolent or admirable personality traits generously mixed in with their bad aspects and so have rich moral character; but for other mad scientists, the good traits are either neglected or greatly abbreviated so that these persons are relatively depraved. This is not a sharp division between good guys and bad guys. It is a more subtle distinction between bad guys whose character is tempered by good traits and bad guys whose good traits are negligible. And so the critical question is, In what circumstances are the good traits of mad scientists well represented, and when are those traits negligible?

The answer is not opaque. One of the first principles in comparing literature with film is that literature commonly describes and develops intentions, remorse, reflections, and maturity, plus other states of mind, much more thoroughly than does film. A text, whether fiction or nonfiction, can use an unlimited vocabulary of words and combinations of words to depict interior feelings. The intangible qualities of moral character—intention, remorse, reflection, maturity—are not more difficult to depict than concrete images. In fact, a reader ordinarily expects a work of fiction to describe the characters' feelings quite thoroughly.

But the means of expression in the medium of film are much more limited. Except for dialogue, music, and sound effects, a film communicates by presenting concrete visual scenes. Emotions and the intangible qualities of moral character must be translated into visual idioms, for example, gestures, facial expressions, and action.[4] The filmmaker must externalize the internal, so to speak. In the words of Edward Murray, "Because he employs a linguistic medium, the novelist is uniquely privileged to explore thoughts and feelings. . . . While some recent film-makers have sought to compete with literature by projecting involved subjective relationships, the cinema possesses a relative weakness in this area."[5]

Three structural differences between fiction and film are especially profound: point of view, manipulation of time, and pace of communication. Nine out of ten films assume "an omniscient and impersonal point of view, regardless of the viewpoint of the novel," says Lester Asheim.[6] Successful experiments in multiple or subjective point of view are rare. Even the greatest such film, Akira Kurosawa's *Rashomon,* must place its four subjective testimonies within an objective frame of reference defined by the time and place of the bandit's trial. By contrast, it is perfectly common for fiction to manipulate point of view with subjunctive moods, conditional tenses, and multiple narrators. A good example is Robert Louis Stevenson's *The Strange Case of Dr. Jekyll and Mr. Hyde,* wherein the reader moves from the point of view of a gentleman, to that of Jekyll's lawyer, to that of Jekyll's medical colleague, and finally to that of Henry Jekyll himself, thus proceeding from the objective observations of the most distant person to the inner feelings of the most anguished one. Film may be capable of doing the same, but the result would be very confusing to the viewer, so almost all cinematic versions of *Jekyll and Hyde* simplify the point of view by rearranging the narrative into a linear sequence. This, incidentally, is a pattern running parallel to that of good television, which I described in chapter 4: as television must greatly simplify its visual imagery, so film must do the same to its narrative structure.

Time receives similar treatment. In film it is almost always condensed to achieve unity of action.[7] Although film can use dissolves and other transitions to bracket scenes of the past, like flashbacks and dreams, those scenes are then depicted with the same cinematic techniques as the present itself.[8] In other words, film lacks a grammar of the past tense, which every written language has.[9] Consider how Mary Shelley's *Frankenstein* tells the story of the creature as a series of flashbacks within the story of the scientist, which is a series of flashbacks within the story of Walton the narrator, which is a series of flashbacks. A Frankenstein film that faithfully replicated this narrative structure would soon have quite a bewildered audience.

Then there is pace. With a text, the reader can pause—between chapters, paragraphs, wherever—to think about the personalities of the characters. Savoring the text is one of the pleasures of reading, so it is well worth the author's effort to give his or her characters some rich personalities. But with film, the viewer has no such control over pace unless he or she is using a videocassette recorder. The viewer receives a film at its own pace, with no opportunity to pause, let alone to savor the work. There is much less reason to dwell on the richness of personalities and much more reason to emphasize action, which keeps the plot moving. And so, says Ingmar Bergman, "the irrational dimension which is the heart of a literary work is often untranslatable" from text to film.[10]

I trust that the implications are obvious. The mad scientists who come to life on the printed page are relatively rich characters, whereas those on the screen are generally more shallow. The audiences that met mad scientists through the texts of Gothic horror often found some personality traits to appreciate, but the audiences that encounter scientists in the cinema see much more simplistic personifications of the evil of science, even if they bear the same names as their literary referents: Frankenstein, Jekyll, Moreau. When the adaptation process begins with a text-to-stage adaptation, as happened with Frankenstein and Jekyll, then the stage versions represent the beginning of simplistic rendering of the mad scientists' depravity.

Subsequent to text-to-film adaptation, there is a second process that also changes the moral character of mad scientists, making them even worse. This is the process of sequels: the *Return of . . . , Son of . . . ,* and *Revenge of . . .* films. The featured attraction in such stories is not the title character of the mad scientist but rather the violent monster, the diabolical invention, or the special visual effect, such as invisibility. The mad scientist or his successor must appear in the film to animate the real attraction, but he has little role thereafter. He becomes more or less interchangeable with his successors. As such he is a cipher who neither requires nor possesses much moral character. Thus, the process of serialization further debases mad scientists by making them more shallow.

By way of illustration, let us consider the series of Invisible Man films. The first, in 1933, was *The Invisible Man,* adapted from the H. G. Wells novel. It told the story of Dr. Jack Griffin, who discovered "monocaine," a drug that made his body invisible but also made him insane. "To make the world grovel at [his] feet," he planned to intimidate humanity by committing murders while invisible.[11] A mad scientist indeed!

In 1940, the Griffin family revisited the invisibility business in *The Return of the Invisible Man,* with Dr. Frank Griffin replacing his brother Jack. Two years later, another Dr. Griffin, grandson of the original Dr. Jack Griffin, activated the invisibility effect in *Invisible Agent.* Two years after that, Dr. Robert Griffin was the title character of *The Revenge of the Invisible Man.*[12] The Griffin name had become a cipher for the science of invisibility by 1944. Finally, Dr. Philip Gray was the scientist in *Abbott and Costello Meet the Invisible Man,* in 1950, and in *The Invisible Man* of 1975, the scientist was Dr. Daniel Weston.[13] Invisibility was the star attraction, and it had a long career, but it only needed interchangeable ciphers of mad scientists after the first film in the series.

To restate my thesis: the moral character of mad scientists, as portrayed in fiction and film, has been changing, both in the process of text-to-film adaptation and in the process of film sequelization. The pattern is that a mad scientist becomes madder as the adaptation process, whether text to stage or text to film, sheds much of the intangible quality of moral character from the text, and he becomes even more shallow as the sequel process reduces him to a succession of ciphers who play perfunctory roles. Ironically, this kind of moral deterioration cannot be attributed to a sustained intellectual critique of science, even though each mad scientist story is an individual critique of scientists or scientific knowledge. Rather, the two processes of moral deterioration have their sources in the art of making films. To illustrate my thesis, let us investigate the two greatest mad scientists: Frankenstein and Jekyll.

THE SYMBOLIC CAREER OF DR. FRANKENSTEIN

The Golem was a creature of artificial life from medieval Jewish folklore. In the earlier Golem stories, learned rabbis shaped humanoid beings from clay, then used spiritual wisdom to invest them with life for a righteous purpose. In the most famous Golem story, Rabbi Loew of Prague (a real person who lived in the seventeenth century) made a Golem to protect the Jewish ghetto from anti-Semitic violence. As stories of artificial life, the Golem tales inevitably addressed the theme of "man's conceit in competing with God."[14] The tales were resolved with the rabbi voluntarily returning the Golem to inanimate clay when its mission had been accomplished, thereby acknowledging the limits of the rabbi's authority over life: "The important point here, then, is that these miracle-working Jews, like Loew, always used their powers wisely; they realized that moral responsibility begins, not ends, with creation, and they destroyed their creatures when they threatened to roam beyond their makers' control."[15]

The later Golem stories were anti-Enlightenment commentaries on scientific knowledge about artificial life and death, for their point was that such knowledge was both unholy and dangerous. Impious rabbis created Golems for frivolous reasons such as hewing wood and hauling water. These Golems subsequently turned violent, forcing their makers to end their lives unhappily.[16]

According to Mary Shelley, her novel *Frankenstein; or, The Modern Prometheus* began with discussions about Dr. Erasmus Darwin's scientific experiments and with a dream in which "the pale student of the unhallowed arts . . . put together . . . the hideous phantasm of a man."[17] Shelley's novel was a secular elaboration of the Golem stories, particularly those that condemned amoral scientific knowledge about how to make a Golem.

Shelley's Victor Frankenstein was a young man with much intellectual curiosity but little moral guidance. As a self-educated youth, he read Paracelsus and other alchemists, thereby leading himself into fantasies of "the elixir of life": "The raising of ghosts or devils was a promise liberally accorded by my favorite authors, the fulfillment of which I most eagerly sought; . . . I was . . . floundering desperately in a very slough of multifarious knowledge, guided by an ardent imagination and childish reasoning."[18] When he went to university to study medicine, an intolerant science professor angrily denounced his alchemical beliefs and attempted to purge them by forcing strong doses of modern rationalist science on young Victor. "I was," he said, "required to exchange chimeras of boundless grandeur for realities of little worth."[19]

A second professor solved the relationship with a benign platitude: a student should apply himself to modern rationalist science but should also honor the medieval alchemists as noble pioneers. From this came the worst possible result. Victor Frankenstein acquired the medical skills of modern science, but he retained the values of those who impiously dabbled with the mystery of life. He made a creature and brought it to life. The Frankenstein who made his own creature was a misguided college boy, a callow youth inexperienced in the ways of the world, let alone in the ways of great evil. Although his deed was reprehensible, he had neither the mind nor the maturity of a master criminal.

Shocked by what he had done, he did the most immature thing imaginable: he abandoned his creature, leaving it to roam through Bavaria and Switzerland. The creature acquired more maturity than young Frankenstein himself. It developed an existential personality based on the anguish of being rejected by its human creator. Shortly after it caused two deaths, Frankenstein met his creature face to face and realized that he had to take responsibility for his creation. This was the first great change in the moral character of the scientist. He and the creature agreed that Frankenstein would solve their joint dilemma by making a female companion for the creature, who would then remove himself and his bride from human civilization. From that point on, Mary Shelley's novel assumed the classic tone of the German doppelgänger genre. The creature became an external reflection, an existential mirror, which forced Victor Frankenstein to consider his own thoughts and actions.

Frankenstein began the work of assembling the creature's bride, then realized the likely consequences of his science. Whereas he had formerly hoped that two such creatures would solve the anguish and violence of one, he later realized that the two, male and female, might beget a terrible race of violent monsters. He destroyed the human parts he had collected to make the bride. That triggered the creature to more violence, killing Frankenstein's best friend and, in a macabre exchange, Frankenstein's bride. This at last brought Frankenstein to accept his ultimate responsibility: he would have to destroy the being he had made, regardless of the consequences, even to himself.

Shelley's novel was a progression from foolish irresponsibility, through increasing responsibility for one's actions, to ultimate responsibility. The scientist painfully "realized that moral responsibility begins, not ends, with creation," as Friedman says of the Golem makers.[21] Although the book was generously laced with evil and violence, their ultimate source was neither the creature nor the scientist. Rather, scientific knowledge, which was both inherently dangerous and powerfully seductive, generated the crimes that punctuated this tale. As the scientist began his story, he cautioned the narrator to "learn from me, if not by my precepts, at least by my example, how dangerous is the acquirement of knowledge."[22] Later in his deathbed testament, Frankenstein echoed that same feeling: "Seek happiness in tranquility and avoid ambition, even if it be only the apparently innocent one of distinguishing yourself in science and discoveries."[23]

The novel appeared in 1818. Five years later an adaptation brought it to the London stage, with the title *Presumption; or, the Fate of Frankenstein*. The shift from the text to stage gave greater prominence to the part of the creature, who stole the show with its sensational appearance and violent actions and who was not humanized through existential anguish.[24] This and later stage versions reduced the narrative to the creation, the bridal scene, and the creature's destruction: "Much of the abstract and philosophical language had to go, as well as the probing into the psyches of Victor and the Monster."[25] The play's judgment of Frankenstein's moral character was a simplistic denunciation of intellectual curiosity, as indicated by the playbill: "The striking moral exhibited in this story is the fatal consequence of that presumption which attempts to penetrate, beyond prescribed depths, into the mysteries of nature."[26]

Three silent films brought Frankenstein to the cinema early in the twentieth century. One of them, the Edison Company's *Frankenstein,* included the doppelgänger theme by showing Frankenstein looking into a mirror and seeing his creature.[27] When James Whale created a new Frankenstein, in 1931, he radically changed the narrative, the characters, and their moral message. Universal Studios commissioned Whale to put the Mary Shelley novel on the screen via a screenplay by Garrett Fort and Francis Faragoh, from an adaptation by John Balderston of a 1927 play by Peggy Webling, plus an independent synopsis by Robert Florey.[28] There were so many intermediate concepts between the novel and the film that fidelity of adaptation was compromised much more than usual. Frankenstein became *Doctor* Frankenstein. From Robert Weine's *The Cabinet of Dr. Caligari* and Paul Wegener's *The Golem* came details of the physical appearance of the creature. From Fritz Lang's *Metropolis* came inspiration for depicting the creation scene as an electrical experiment rather than a chemical process.[29]

Frankenstein's science was ungodly: he demanded human cadavers, no matter where or how. And "Herr Frankenstein was interested only in human life—first to destroy it, then recreate it. There you have his mad dream!"[30]

Dr. Frankenstein was arrogant, reckless, and hysterical, preventing any bond of empathy between the audience and himself. It was a different scientist, Professor Waldman, who decided to destroy the creature. (While Waldman did that, Frankenstein went home to prepare for his wedding.) Thus, Frankenstein was removed from responsibility for his own acts. The creature-as-doppelgänger, which in the novel had nurtured the scientist's sense of responsibility, was absent from the film. The creature was slightly humanized, but mostly its role was to keep the film exciting by supplying violence upon violence. So, too, the creature's violence was explained in terms of the blunder of Fritz the assistant, who brought the brain of a criminal ("Dysfunctio Cerebri," said the label) to be inserted into the creature's head. Dr. Frankenstein's isolation from civilization and its moral influence was extreme. "At night the winds howl in the mountains," he wrote. "There is no one here. Prying eyes can't peer into my secret."[31]

James Whale's *Frankenstein* represented all the best and all the worst of horror films. Suspense, emotion, violence, and counterviolence combined to make a thrilling story, yet they also inflicted their inevitable damage on the moral character of the mad scientist. Whereas in the novel Frankenstein's intentions were somewhat naive, in the film they were purely arrogant: to humble the scientists who had denounced his work. As to remorse and responsibility, Dr. Frankenstein delegated them to Dr. Waldman. Much of the novel concerned Frankenstein's interior turmoil, but the fast-paced film allowed him no time to reflect on himself. The scientist's level of maturity was especially changed, from Victor Frankenstein's college-boy folly to Dr. Henry Frankenstein's careful planning based on much scientific experience. In all three features of moral character, the mad scientist who represented the evil of science was distinctly more depraved in the film than in the novel.

Then it got worse in the sequels. *The Bride of Frankenstein,* which Whale made for Universal in 1935, first presented Dr. Henry Frankenstein as a remorseful penitent: "I have been cursed for delving into the mysteries of Life—perhaps Death is sacred, and I have profaned it."[32] Very soon, however, he subordinated himself to Dr. Septimus Pretorius, his evil mentor from the medical college. Pretorius controlled Henry Frankenstein by controlling the monster, to whom he promised a monster-wife, and by kidnapping Frankenstein's wife, Elizabeth. This ultradiabolical scientist who robbed graves and, like Paracelsus himself, grew homunculi in bell jars, was more frightening than Frankenstein.

In *Son of Frankenstein,* Dr. Wolf von Frankenstein, the title character, reanimated the creature. The doctor foolishly ignored the warnings of the simple peasants and underestimated the creature's violence. Now the creature was controlled not by this Dr. Frankenstein but by Ygor, the crippled grave robber. In effect, the scientist was a spectator to the moral conflicts of his scientific research.

In *The Ghost of Frankenstein,* Dr. Ludwig Frankenstein, brother of Wolf, son of Henry, experimented on the creature. His brash intentions, however, were subverted by Dr. Theodor Bohmer, an evil mentor much like Dr. Septimus Pretorius. Bohmer tricked Dr. Frankenstein into putting Ygor's brain into the creature, with the result that "I've created a hundred times the Monster that my father made!"[33]

Subsequent monster-resuscitators in the Universal series were Dr. Frank Mannerling, assisted by Elsa Frankenstein (daughter of Ludwig, granddaughter of Henry) in *Frankenstein Meets the Wolfman;* Dr. Gustav Niemann (lunatic and graverobber) in *House of Frankenstein;* Dr. Frantz Edelmann in *House of Dracula;* and Dr. Sandra Mornay in *Abbott and Costello Meet Frankenstein.* All were either evil from the beginning, or they quickly sank into depravity when scientific glory seduced them.

Ironically, this tradition also includes a series of films that treated the moral character of Frankenstein as a rich moral personality. This was the Hammer group directed by Terence Fisher and starring Peter Cushing. *The Curse of Frankenstein,* released in 1957, shifted the center of interest away from the monster and back to the scientist.[34] He was indeed blasphemous: a grave robber, a murderer, and a maker of artificial life, but at the same time, "a magnificently arrogant aristocratic rebel, in the direct Byron tradition."[35]

The following year his dual personality received even closer attention, with no distractions from any monsters, in *The Revenge of Frankenstein.* Dr. Frankenstein was a most compassionate and dedicated surgeon, but then he used his position to amputate recklessly and steal the separated parts for the purpose of healing a pitiful hunchback by making a new body for him. Which was the real character of Frankenstein, and how should we assess it? Was he the hypocritical but much-appreciated surgeon or the much-reviled, yet altruistic scientist? Fisher forced this question on his audiences but permitted no easy answers. David Pirie comments, "The sadistic and noble elements in [Frankenstein's] character thus exist side by side."[36]

Next of the Fisher-Cushing films was *Frankenstein Created Woman.* Again the namesake scientist did a most ungodly thing but for the goodliest of reasons. To retrieve some goodness from the tragic deaths of the lovers Christina and Hans, Dr. Frankenstein transplanted the soul of Hans into the body of Christina, thus uniting them in artificial life, cheating the afterlife, and surgically creating transsexuality.

Lastly there was *Frankenstein Must Be Destroyed.* For his repertoire of evil habits, there were murder, kidnapping, and blackmail. For his good work—embedded in evil habits—he saved the brain of a fellow scientist by transplanting it into another person's body. Unfortunately, the old brain hated its new existence. Should Frankenstein have done this? "The audience is again being forced to make a complex moral judgment about Frankenstein's character and actions. He has performed a grotesque operation on his colleague and yet we know that he has saved his life and his sanity."[37]

In those four films, Dr. Frankenstein had much evil in him, but his evil was tempered by uncertain quantities of goodness. He intrigued his viewers, perhaps also won their sympathy, and, let us hope, left them thinking about how each person balances the good and evil within.[38] In the more typical films of the Frankenstein legend, however, the personality of the scientist was greatly abbreviated. Instead of asking questions about character, most such films presented the scientist as a simplistic symbol of the evil of science. This was especially acute in the later Universal films, wherein the monster needed only a cipher of a scientist to ignite its violence.

THE SYMBOLIC AND SEXUAL CAREER OF DR. JEKYLL

Robert Louis Stevenson was long worried about the duality of human nature. During his youth in Scotland, the forces of Calvinist and Victorian morality persuaded him that beneath the surface of goodness and propriety was a realm of chaos and violence, so that one's life was a constant conflict between the two levels.

According to the plot of *The Strange Case of Dr. Jekyll and Mr. Hyde,* published in 1886, a respectable scientist released the evil personality within himself. At first he enjoyed the pleasures of the dark self, but then he recognized the consequences, regretted his experiments, and attempted to suppress the evil character. He struggled to regain his own good worth, but ultimately his experiment led to his destruction. He did recover his moral bearings before he died, and he had a reservoir of moral strength to struggle heroically against his evil half.

Stevenson depicted Jekyll's initial goodness in terms of altruistic intent. If the good and the evil sides of the human personality "could but be housed in separate identities, life would be relieved of all that was unbearable. . . . The just could walk steadfastly and securely on his upward path, doing the good things in which he found his pleasure, and no longer exposed to disgrace and penitence by the hands of this extraneous evil. It was the curse of mankind that these incongruous faggots were thus bound together. . . . How, then, were they dissociated?"[39]

When Jekyll succeeded in splitting the two selves, he fell into depravity by indulging the Hyde personality. "I knew myself, at the first breath of this new life, to be more wicked, tenfold more wicked, sold as a slave to my original evil."[40] But then he became profoundly re-morseful after Hyde wantonly murdered a man. According to the au-thor, "Henry Jekyll, with streaming tears of gratitude and remorse, had fallen upon his knees and lifted his clasped hands to God. . . . Hyde was henceforth impossible; whether I would or not, I was now con-fined to the better part of my existence; and, oh, how I rejoiced to think it! With what willing humility I embraced anew the restrictions of natural life."[41]

From that point on, Jekyll struggled mightily to suppress the per-sonality of Hyde. Unfortunately, the cumulative effects of the trans-forming drug caused Hyde to arise again despite Jekyll's remorse. As the power of Hyde increased, so did the moral sensitivity of Jekyll, but eventually the Hyde personality overcame Jekyll.

When this story was adapted for the stage in 1887, a romantic interest, a girlfriend for Jekyll, was added.[42] Now Stevenson's dual-personality theme could take the tangible form of a contrast between Jekyll's chaste behavior and Hyde's lust. Stevenson objected to this sexual interpretation, but it nevertheless became fixed into the vari-ous dramatic productions.[43] Between 1908 and 1920, there were about a dozen silent film versions. The 1912 film by the Thanhauser com-pany divided the romantic interest into two women, with Jekyll torn between them.[44] The 1920 version, starring John Barrymore, contin-ued this sexual interpretation by emphasizing the difference between Millicent, the proper lady, and Gina, the dance-hall prostitute who be-came Hyde's mistress. Carlos Clarens remarks, "The introduction of the latter [Gina] . . . serves to expand the character of Hyde from the child-beating murderer of the original into a more sexually complex personality."[45]

Not surprisingly, sex made things different. At first the romantic relations gave more substance to the dual-personality theme in the contrast between chastity and lust. But later they subverted this theme when opinions on sexual ethics changed: Jekyll's sexuality should not have been repressed in the first place, and Hyde's sexuality was an understandable solution to Jekyll's sexual needs.

The next major work, Rouben Mamoulian's 1932 *Dr. Jekyll and Mr. Hyde,* starring Fredric March, was made at a time when the Ameri-can public was newly fascinated by Sigmund Freud's theories on sexu-ality and hysteria. Never mind that those theories were often misunderstood. The point is that for much of the public, a wide range of human behavior could be clinically explained in terms of sexual tension, uncomplicated by moral judgment.

In this film Dr. Henry Jekyll had a fiancée named Muriel Carew. Their prim and proper engagement constituted love without sex. Jekyll then encountered an attractive prostitute named Ivy Pearson, and he used his transforming drug to become Hyde so that he could have a lusty affair with Ivy. Whereas the life of Jekyll, particularly his relations with Muriel, constituted a world of propriety, discipline, and sexual repression, the life of Hyde was a hearty escape from those unhappy bonds.[46] By this reasoning, the audience could hardly blame Jekyll for becoming Hyde.

From his first meeting with Ivy, Jekyll was a prisoner of his own sexuality. The two murders he committed as Hyde were entwined in his lust for Ivy. Before that Muriel was to blame for his sexual frustration. In other words, Dr. Jekyll was not responsible for his own actions, according to the popular interpretation of Freudian theory that guided this film. Thus, much of the "moral argument and explicit comment" of Stevenson's narrative were eliminated.[47] Jekyll did not become more evil in the film. Rather, his moral character mattered much less in the nonjudgmental version of pop Freudianism.

Although there were "Son of Dr. Jekyll" and a "Daughter of Dr. Jekyll" sequels, most of the dozens of remakes preserved the person of the original doctor but then interpreted his personality in new ways. In *The Two Faces of Dr. Jekyll,* directed by Terence Fisher for Hammer in 1961, the doctor was a dull married man whose wife was having an affair. When Jekyll turned himself into Hyde, he consorted with a dance-hall prostitute and also discovered his wife's infidelity. Subsequently, he used the person of Hyde to murder the wife's lover and rape his own wife.[48] This sequence of events entirely reversed the Jekyll-Hyde relationship as posited by Stevenson. In the original, Hyde eventually controlled the relationship and Jekyll succumbed, but in the 1961 film Jekyll controlled it and manipulated Hyde, both to enjoy his own sexuality and punish his wife's.

The most bizarre sexual interpretation of Jekyll and Hyde also came from Hammer. This was *Dr. Jekyll and Sister Hyde,* directed by Roy Ward Baker in 1971. The scientist's potion became contaminated with sex hormones, so that Jekyll transformed himself into a woman and pretended to be his own sister. With his transexuality-in-a-jar, he was able to expand his love life to include both a man's and a woman's experiences.

One more point of reference: in David Wickes's *Jekyll and Hyde,* broadcast on American television in January 1990, Jekyll was a widower who became involved with his married sister-in-law. In the form of Jekyll he rejected her advances, but in the form of Hyde he brutally raped her. Yet when he explained the Jekyll-Hyde connection to her, she forgave his actions. It seems to me that this was the most extreme equivocation of sexual ethics in the entire Jekyll-and-Hyde tradition, for it suggested that a brutal rape was excusable on the grounds that the rapist and the victim really loved each other.

Whereas Stevenson had described moral duality in terms of a very clear struggle between Jekyll's character and Hyde's depravity, the sexual interpretation of Jekyll and Hyde gradually subverted that duality and erased its clarity. When Hyde became the outlet for Jekyll's sexual needs, he was no longer Jekyll's moral opposite. Rather, he became an extension of Jekyll's personality. When social standards of sexual behavior became more tolerant, and sexual repression lost the legitimacy it had enjoyed in the climate of Victorian values, then the transition back and forth between Jekyll and Hyde lacked the opprobrium that Stevenson had intended. I do not mean that all sexual themes are dangerous. But in the case of Dr. Henry Jekyll, the sequence of highly subjective sexual interpretations subverted the firm platform of moral duality upon which Stevenson's scientist discovered his own good character and asserted it heroically. Why he struggled against Hyde and how he did so were altered. Previously he had felt profound remorse for his crimes and sins and then had accepted responsibility for them, attempting to contain the evil he had unleashed. More recently, his relation to Hyde has been released from moral judgment, whether favorable or not. The ethical ambiguity of Jekyll's modern sex life prevents him from acting out the exercise in moral character that Stevenson intended.

THE ARTISTIC LIFE OF SYMBOLS

Powerful currents of hostility surround the institution of science, and stories of mad scientists, whether textual or cinematic, constitute an extremely effective anti-Enlightenment vehicle for conveying those sentiments. They thrill their audiences by brewing together suspense, horror, violence, and heroism and by uniting those features under the premise that most scientists are dangerous. Untrue, perhaps; preposterous, perhaps; lowbrow, perhaps, but nevertheless effective.

We must look into the dark heart of Gothic horror to understand how it commissions its mad scientists to tell the world that science is evil. One way to interpret its fiction and film is to posit a real-life referent and then dissect the work of art as a slight variation on reality. *Dr. Strangelove,* for example, elicits a parlor game in which friends can argue whether the title character is based on Wernher von Braun, Edward Teller, Herman Kahn, Henry Kissinger, or someone else. In other words, cultural images of science are derived from social realities of science. In this view, mad scientist stories are close copies of the actual evils of science. But if that were true of mad scientist stories in general, then their increasing depravity would indicate that most real scientists have become increasing depraved and that someone like Josef Mengele owns a part of each scientist's soul.

The other style of interpretation is to locate these symbols of the evil of science in artistic processes that operate more or less independently of real science and real scientists. It suggests that text-to-stage and text-to-film adaptation, plus serialization, accounts for the increasing depravity of the mad scientist stories.

In the previous four chapters, I began with certain cultural meanings and then asked how symbols of science arose to give them flesh-and-blood expression. I implied that the work of the symbols depended on the needs of their respective meanings: symbols in the service of meanings, so to speak. The case of the mad scientists also involves symbols serving meanings, but then it adds a twist. Little changes in these symbols can cause big changes in their respective cultural meanings: adaptation and serialization greatly intensify the feeling that science is evil. Meanings are somewhat vulnerable to artistic capricity in the construction of symbols.

If the personality of Dr. Frankenstein symbolizes science, and that personality loses the good traits it once had; if the moral character of Dr. Jekyll embodies the same thing, and its heroic qualities are replaced by moral ambiguity; if the process of moral deterioration comes from the art of making stories, then the changes in this device for damning science deserve to be understood.

Technically, text-to-film adaptation is no worse for mad scientists than for cowboys in Westerns or lovers in romances. But the moral consequences are exceptional. There are some bad guys in the other two genres, but Westerns do not condemn cowboy life in general, and romances are not usually dedicated to the theme that love is evil. Because mad scientist stories are indeed condemnations of rationalist science, and because the personality of the scientist is the principal symbol of the evil of science, any change in his personality is likely to change the critique. If his moral character worsens because of adaptation or serialization, then so does the moral character of science itself, as posited by a particular narrative.

Historically, this dynamic means that the antirationalist critique of science became harsher in nineteenth-century stage adaptations than in the original prose. The critique was harsher still when films were launched from the stage adaptations, creating definitive cinematic personalities for Doctors Frankenstein, Jekyll, Griffin, Moreau, and others. After that, most of their sequels further simplified their moral character, which further debased the moral worth of science as measured by these movies.

If artistic processes have made mad scientists much more depraved, then regardless of how moral or immoral scientists actually are, the symbolic careers of Doctors Frankenstein, Jekyll, Caligari et al. are particularly worrisome, for their source is independent of scientific reality. In fact, this problem is like a runaway Golem. Scientists may have inspired it, but they cannot control it.

PART FOUR

■ ■ ■

*Conjuring
Science*

CHAPTER TEN

■ ■ ■

A Manual for Conjurers

Earlier I offered an anthropological model of science in American life: cultural meanings acquire a semblance of being scientific as the symbols of science are detached from the intellectual substance of science and then reattached to those meanings. The usual symbols of science—curvaceous microscopes, humming computer screens, latinate diplomas, and images such as that of the cold fusion flask—are vulnerable to being expropriated by causes and ideologies that have little or nothing to do with science. The result is that various movements, parties, and interest groups can bestow the plenary authority of science on their own private meanings. With a little creativity in the art of conjuring, any group can make its views seem scientific.

After having seen that model illustrated in five episodes, and perhaps after you, my reader, have recalled other episodes that illustrate the same model, we can see some patterns arising. Now we can gather those patterns into a descriptive model of the same thing, that is, a menu of tricks for conjuring science.

My descriptive model comprises nine observations on science in American life. The first four are statements about the cultural conditions that make it possible to conjure science. Together they provide a general framework within which we can consider more specific observations. The next two observations concern scientific authority and personal credentials. The last three address issues of knowledge and certainty.

I begin with framework observations: Whichever way we define science—a social institution, a body of knowledge, a package of values, or an intellectual process—we should realize that nonscientists have strong feelings about science, but we cannot expect their feelings to be anchored in scientists' definitions of science. People project their own extrinsic cultural meanings onto science, and they seem to appreciate science to the degree that it confirms their own values. These meanings and values are not necessarily antiscientific or pseudoscientific. They are only extrascientific in the sense that they do not answer to such formal scientific values as rationalism, naturalism, secularism, or science for the sake of science.

We can see this projection happening repeatedly, as when the science of fluoridation is equated with soul-snatching (at which point the science of *anti*fluoridation becomes a virtue of heroic resistance), when some medical knowledge of AIDS/HIV becomes a platform for an apocalyptic-authoritarian political model, or when a little faith in cold fusion sustains a lot of faith in simplistic solutions to our energy problems. Likewise, when evolutionary thought is charged with being a theory of moral anarchy or when an anti-Enlightenment theory about evil takes the form of scientists in fiction and film.

This process may be unsettling, but it is not necessarily sinister. For many thousands of years, other human institutions, including religion, politics, and art, have had extrinsic values projected onto them, thereby subverting both the integrity of internal values and the clarity of internal knowledge. Even if this process is less than desirable, our institutions survive it.

In the case of science in American culture, Charles Rosenberg describes this phenomenon—that people project their own extrinsic cultural meanings onto science—better than anyone else, so I call this phenomenon "Rosenberg's Observation."[1]

If that observation portrays a tension between intrinsic and extrinsic values, then it also raises a historical question: how did this tension come about? After all, the Protestant model of nature and science suffered no such tension for a century or more, until the arrival of the European scientific research ethos. The philosophy of useful knowledge used to harmonize popular values, with scientific values, and it still does. Where, then, does the tension come from?

"Burnham's and LaFollette's Observation" answers this question: the process of popularizing the new scientific ethos separated public understanding from expert understanding by trivializing public knowledge about that ethos.[2] Even though this process began more than one hundred years ago, its habits and its effects continue today in the form of mediocre science education and sensationalist journalism. Science then becomes a series of wonders, miracles, or life-and-death melodramas. The effect of this process has been to break up the public's understanding of science into a fragmented miscellany of trivia, mystery, and trinkets ("snippets without context") unrelated to such habits as empiricism or the hypothetico-deductive method.[3]

This effect brings us to a peculiar status quo. American citizens respect science as a kind of religion in the sense that it supposedly has a plenary authority to answer all of our questions and to solve all of our problems. But a screen of mysterious symbols comes between the citizen and the intellectual substance of science. Esoteric experts and the abracadabra of technical jargon are the modern-day burning bushes and pillars of fire. Elsewhere I called this science in an Old Testament style. Now permit me to call this "Toumey's Observation."

None of this matters very much if the life of science proceeds apart from the rest of American life. If our scientists make themselves happy without regard to the feelings or the values or the fears of other Americans, which is to say that if the moral autonomy of science is a realistic theory about science and society, then no one should lose any sleep over Rosenberg's Observation, Burnham's and LaFollette's Observation, or Toumey's Observation. But those three observations become serious indeed to the degree that American democratic culture demands that science and scientists answer to the common values and themes of American life. And that is exactly the point of democratic science, as I described it in chapter 3. I also call this "Larson's Observation" because I derive my core views on democratic science from the comments of Edward Larson.[4]

Larson's Observation is especially evident when a town decides by direct popular vote whether to fluoridate its water or when a state, such as California, resolves its policies on AIDS/HIV by the same kind of mechanism. It is also evident in other procedures of democratic culture: government decisions to give millions of dollars to research on cold fusion, as an exercise in the virtue of hope, and local school board decisions to teach creationism as science, as a reaction against the supposed moral anarchy embodied in evolutionary thought.

Within the framework of these four general observations, we can consider some of the specific habits by which American culture treats science and scientists. Here I identify two patterns by which the abstract institutional authority of science is realized in the personal credibility of individual scientists.

There is, says Gary Downey, a "systematic ambiguity in the public identities of scientists in American culture."[5] As an abstract entity, the institution of science is a powerful authority, but individual scientists begin with zero credibility when they represent particular positions in a dispute. They endure a constant burden of establishing and defending their own personal scientific credibility. The usual way to do so is to cobble together a suitable simulacrum of personal credibility from the standard symbols (Ph.D.s, quantities of publications, faculty titles, and so on), while trying to deny their adversaries the same credibility.

To be candid, this task may not be particularly difficult. In *The Imaginary Invalid,* Molière writes "You have but to hold forth in cap and gown, and any gibberish becomes learning, all nonsense passes for sense."[6] The more recent version of the same thing is known as the Doctor Fox Effect. An actor who knew nothing about a particular scientific topic memorized a script about it, and he used his acting skills to deliver a lecture to an audience of well-educated professionals. The majority judged him "stimulating and interesting"; one person in the audience claimed to have read an article written by this Dr. Fox. "The researchers [who arranged this demonstration] concluded that even well-educated audiences cannot necessarily detect propaganda or false information."[7]

We can name this relationship between institutional authority and an individual's credibility "Downey's Observation": each scientist has to establish her or his personal connection to the institutional authority of science. Downey's Observation may be amusing in the case of Molière's physician and the apocryphal Doctor Fox, but it was not so funny when public health officials had their professional integrity challenged in ad hominem attacks from Lyndon LaRouche's cohorts in the 1986 campaign on Proposition 64.

Neither is it humorous when scientists face essentially frivolous charges of scientific misconduct, as in the cases of Paul Fisher, Herbert Needleman, and Erdem Cantekin. Fisher studied cigarette advertising aimed at children, Needleman researched children's exposure to lead, and Cantekin tested the use of amoxicillin, a common antibiotic, as a treatment for children's inner-ear infections. In each of these cases, the scientist's conclusions threatened the interests of the relevant industry. In each of these cases, the scientist was subsequently accused of professional misconduct. In each, the scientist's conduct and conclusions were eventually vindicated. In the meantime, however, Fisher, Needleman, and Cantekin had to endure long, miserable, time-consuming investigations.[8]

I want to add a second observation on individual scientists and institutional authority. Our media, both print and electronic, typically present a scientific dispute as a two-sided matter by giving both sides approximately equal time or space to state their views and criticize their opponents' views. This might be because our altruistic media cannot help but love fairness, but I think it is more likely that a juicy tit-for-tat argument makes a good story. (In addition, television and radio are required to a certain extent to let people respond to attacks by giving them airtime.)

This habit of the media leads to a systematic distortion of scientific authority when one scientist representing a small faction of dissidents or insurgents receives as much media attention as another scientist representing the majority of experts in that field, for equal time makes it *seem* that the scientific community is about equally divided when it is not. I call this phenomenon the "pseudosymmetry of scientific authority." It was evident in the fluoridation controversies when one antifluoridationist dentist in a community could negate the strong professional consensus of almost all other dentists by virtue of the media giving both sides equal time. So, too, it could be seen in the 1986 campaigns for and against the LaRouche Initiative whenever California talk shows reduced the question to a one on-one debate between representatives of both sides.

This phenomenon has also been evident in the creation-evolution controversies of the past three decades. Creationists have repeatedly suggested that the scientific consensus on evolution is disintegrating, and they have implied that large proportions of the scientific community are currently becoming creationists. Neither of those contentions is accurate. Nevertheless, Justice Antonin Scalia of the U.S. Supreme Court, in his dissenting opinion on the case of Louisiana's creationism law, took those creationist claims at face value. "The [creationist] witnesses," he wrote, "repeatedly assured committee members [of the Louisiana legislature] that 'hundreds and hundreds' of highly respected, internationally renowned scientists believed in creation science and would support their testimony."[9]

According to one group of researchers, this pattern of behavior "conveys . . . the notion that one side is as credible as the other. . . . But often one side represents mainstream scientific thought, while the other is a minority of dissident voices. . . . It is deceptive to present such opposing positions as if they had equal support."[10] Such is the pseudosymmetry of scientific authority.

My next three observations concern knowledge and certainty. We know that ordinarily most humans need a measure of certainty in their lives, including both factual certainty and moral certainty. In addition, we know that many Americans attribute to science the plenary authority of a religion, which means that they expect to find some certainty in science. Such an expectation is wrong-minded, in my view, because it confuses two institutions, science and religion, which are both legitimate but are also legitimately different. Nevertheless, science should give us certainty, both factual and moral, according to the feelings of many citizens. From this feeling comes a simple moral standard for judging scientific knowledge: it is natural, right, and proper for knowledge to take the form of certainty, but it is highly disturbing—unnatural—for science to conclude that our knowledge of a given problem is riddled with uncertainty. Candor about uncertainty is not what people want.

This brings us to the heavy weight of a little uncertainty. When scientific conclusions are less than certain, they are considered less than scientific. Furthermore, a little bit of uncertainty equals a very large proportion of doubt about the scientific validity of a given conclusion. Many people have noted this, but Benjamin Paul put this insight into words very well in the case of the fluoridation controversies, so I name it "Paul's Observation."[11] Epidemiologists and other public heath officials were very confident that fluoridating water was a good idea, but none of them could say honestly to a degree of 100 percent certainty that no one would ever suffer an adverse reaction to fluoride. This little splinter of uncertainty then became a large plank of the ideological opposition to fluoride.

Paul's observation has a corollary. Replicable demonstrations of cause and effect, in experimental conditions, are the stuff of scientific certainty, but conclusions derived from statistical probability are less than scientific because they are, by definition, less than certain. Almost every statistical description of an interesting phenomenon, no matter how powerful it is statistically, is less than 100 percent certain. We can see Paul's Observation and its corollary in the tobacco industry's stance on smoking and disease, which describes the connection between smoking and cancer as possible but not certain, in which case nicotine addicts have a mechanism for discounting all the statistical evidence on smoking and disease.

Paul's Observation must be especially disheartening to epidemiologists. Ideally, their discipline merges statistical surveys with replicable test-tube demonstrations of biological cause and effect, but typically survey research moves much faster than laboratory work, which is to say that epidemiology's *uncertain* knowledge is ahead of its certain knowledge. Gary Taubes points to a serious historical problem in this field. Epidemiologists have successfully discovered and described the most statistically powerful associations of behavior and disease, like smoking and cancer, or of environment and disease, like secondhand smoke and cancer, in which case they are now left with phenomena that are statistically marginal, at best, like electromagnetic fields and leukemia.[12] If a little bit of uncertainty equals a very large proportion of doubt, then a lot of uncertainty equals pure incredulity.

Next is "Mazur's Observation": public reaction against a given technology increases in proportion to media reports about it, even when those reports are carefully balanced. Allan Mazur notices this in the cases of fluoridation and nuclear power.[13] It seems that technology is equated with change, change with uncertainty, and uncertainty with risk. Risk, of course, demands caution. This is not to say that the media create those feelings. Instead, Mazur implies, those feelings are commonplace, but dormant, until media coverage of a given story about technology brings them back to the surface. Even if media coverage is not particularly critical, it still raises fears about the technology it describes.

Finally, there are "reversals of scientific conclusions." According to a common belief, the growth of scientific knowledge is linear and progressive. Yesterday's scientific conclusions constitute a reliable foundation of truth on which today's conclusions rest securely. Then when today's contradict or reverse yesterday's, some people take a morbid delight in the failure of science to meet that ideal expectation, but many more feel disturbed, even betrayed, by the unavoidable realization that science is sometimes wrong and that scientists are imperfect.

This is bad enough as an abstract principle that reflects on science as an impersonal institution, as when information from the Hubble telescope causes astronomers to revise their estimates of the age of the universe. That reversal discredits astronomers, but it is hardly an existential catastrophe to the rest of us. Such reversals of scientific conclusions, however, are far more disturbing when they affect scientific knowledge about medicine and health. People want to enjoy good health, and they want to escape the inevitability of aging. They follow scientific news about health and medicine, and they act on that news. When today's news contradicts yesterday's, they conclude that science has made fools of them.

Consider antioxidants. At one time not very long ago, there was a consensus, uniting both scientists and their public, about the value of vitamins A and E. They prevent cancer, it was believed, because the antioxidants they contain help thwart the mischief of free radicals, which are often implicated in cancer. The consumption of these vitamins became an act of faith in that scientific knowledge. Then in 1994 scientists in Finland reported that heavy smokers who took those vitamins suffered *higher* rates of lung cancer than did heavy smokers who took placebos.[14]

A similar kind of confusion confounds studies of alcohol and cardiovascular health. A recent American study found that moderate drinking in a range of one to three drinks a week was ideal for cardiovascular health, regardless of the kind of alcohol. A Danish study at the same time described the ideal range as three to five drinks *a day,* but only for wine.[15] So which is it—a maximum of three drinks a week or a minimum of twenty-one a week, only wine or any kind of alcohol?

The most confused matter of all, at this writing, is breast cancer. Throughout 1994 and 1995, the subject of breast cancer was clouded with public disagreements about genetic factors versus other putative causes, statistical errors and scientific misconduct, and levels of risk in estrogen replacement therapy. Because this is one of the most common forms of cancer, it is especially tragic that multiple scientific studies yield multiple different conclusions about breast cancer.

Why do these reports reverse and contradict each other? They do so because scientists are human and human knowledge is imperfect. But when scientific knowledge is expected to be more or less certain, which is to say more or less perfect, this kind of knowledge acquires a moral taint. Uncertainty and imperfection must not be taken for granted. Rather, they must be judged as betrayals in the sense that science has deviated, for no good reason, from ideal expectations.

Such are the nine observations in my descriptive model. Think of them like this: the four framework observations constitute a license to conjure science; the next two, on institutional authority and individual credentials, show how to conjure the latter from the former (Downey's Observation) and the former from the latter (the pseudosymmetry of scientific authority); the last three, on knowledge and certainty, show how to transmute scientific knowledge into something better or something worse by depicting it either as a kind of certainty or a kind of uncertainty. This is not far different from the alchemist's ability to turn a base substance into a precious metal or a precious substance into a base metal.

Some of these observations contradict each other. According to Downey's Observation, individual scientists try to derive their personal credibility from the institutional authority of science, but the pseudosymmetry of scientific authority implies that this institutional authority can be reduced to personal credibility. Science is believed to be a transcendental source of moral and factual certainty, as can be inferred from Toumey's Observation, except when a tiny drop of uncertainty or equivocation undermines all the transcendental power of science, as suggested by Paul's Observation and reversals of scientific conclusions. My descriptive model is also incomplete. I invite you to expand, amend, and revise it by raising your own observations and substantiating them in additional episodes of conjured science.

■ ■ ■

Now, I have some loose ends to tie up. I have spoken coarsely of a world divided into scientists and nonscientists and thus have done little justice to various degrees of scientific literacy in between. Nor have I explored such internal categories as race, class, gender, and occupation. I agree that cultural problems have social dimensions, which is to say that sociological knowledge is one of the anthropologist's best friends. But in this book I tilt much more toward cultural issues at the expense of social variables because my intention has been to describe the place of science in American life as a cultural problem, at a synoptic level. I have tried to stay focused on one problem, when the alternative would have been to multiply the length of this book by multiplying the number of problems and issues that *could be* connected to the cultural problem of science in American life. Nevertheless, I hope that my treatment of this cultural problem will help those who want to address the relevant social questions—for instance, sociologists and others who can build on this work by showing how race, class, gender, occupation, or other social variables affect the place of science in American life.

This brings me to a related problem. The social sciences, including anthropology and sociology, are much concerned about questions of power. I am used to other scholars asking about power in a Marxist voice (how do the powerful and the powerless stand in relation to the means of production?) or in a Foucaultian tone (how is knowledge transformed into an impersonal culture of power that dehumanizes everyone?). Like Southerners who place a person by asking, "Where do you go to church?" we place each other by asking, "What is your theory of power?"

I expect to be asked that question, but my answer will disappoint many. My theory about science in American life is not a theory of power. Rather, it is a hermeneutic theory, a story of meanings and symbols, that addresses questions other than those about power.

I recognize that my views on meanings and symbols can intersect with theories of power; power can go to those who best manipulate the symbols of science. Indeed, my account of the campaign in favor of Proposition 64 by Lyndon LaRouche and his followers shows it to have been an obvious exercise in political power, employing some popular symbols of science.

My other case studies, however, are not so simple. No doubt the antifluoridationists' deployment of symbols served their goal of winning referenda. The creationists' construction of a pejorative definition of evolution assisted their campaign to enhance creationism's credibility at the direct expense of evolution's. So hermeneutics intersected with power. But this does not mean that hermeneutics can be reduced to power or even that a thirst for power inspired these two hermeneutic exercises. On the contrary, strong existential currents were the driving forces. The antifluoridationists sincerely felt that the practice of fluoridating water was a real threat to personal integrity, and the creationists truly believed that the idea of evolution was deeply implicated in moral anarchy. When we take into account these existential currents, theories of power are incomplete at best. Remember that the antifluoridationist movement won 60 percent of its referenda, which is surely power. But instead of consolidating that power or continuing to enjoy it, the antifluoridationist movement dissipated as

Americans turned to other existential concerns, indicating that what we label "power" is contingent on what we call "existential."

The other two episodes have even less to do with power. One can say that several people at the University of Utah were motivated by visions of lucrative patent rights and that film studios make mad scientist movies to make money. Such statements are true, but they do not explain the cultural content of either faith in cold fusion or mad scientist stories. Instead, both kinds of content come from long-standing cultural meanings that have little to do with power.

And so I acknowledge that the hermeneutics of science intersects with power *sometimes,* and I invite my readers to consider the intersections. But to keep theories of power in perspective, I insist that in other cases the hermeneutics of science are *not* power-laden, which is to say that these questions of meanings and symbols should not be equated with questions of power.

Another bit of unfinished business is the problem of hermeneutic symmetry. In the episodes I have presented to illustrate my theory, both sides of a controversy ought to be equally interesting for the ways they use symbols to convey meanings. The case for fluoridation should be just as germane as the case against it, the defense of the Orthodox Paradigm of AIDS/HIV deserves as much attention as the attack on it, and the hermeneutics of justifying evolutionary thought ought to be compared with the hermeneutics of trashing that body of thought. But there is a catch: too many scientists believe that science is objective in its methods and conclusions, in which case they use a language of objectivity to communicate their knowledge. They write and speak in a style that suppresses moral, existential, and subjective meaning. The "symbolic strategy" of science, writes Clifford Geertz, "is restrained, spare, resolutely analytic; by shunning the semantic devices that most effectively formulate moral sentiment, it seeks to maximize intellectual clarity."[16] Call this "Geertz's Observation": the intrinsic values of the scientific research ethos disguise the extrinsic cultural turmoil that surrounds it. (See how easy it is to expand my descriptive model?)

The consequence is that both sides are *not* equally interesting hermeneutically. Those who are creative with symbols and meanings, whether scientists or not, have a distinct advantage over those who try to conform to the intellectual purity of the scientific research ethos. In the fluoridation controversies, this helps explain why voters in about one thousand referenda were deeply moved by crusaders who spoke of personal integrity versus soul-snatching and hardly moved at all by authorities who thought that the collective wisdom of epidemiology, biochemistry, and dentistry was self-evident. The same holds for competing views concerning AIDS/HIV: whether it is about an apocalyptic plague, and the moral implications thereof, or about the molecular biology of viruses. This is also true of evolution. Is it a choice between chaos, represented by evolution, and moral order, represented by creationism? Or is it a natural history of Galápagos finches, English pepper moths, and fossil remains with hard-to-pronounce names? Let us disregard, for a moment, our own scientific preferences about fluoridation, AIDS/HIV, and evolution while we consider which side has the more interesting things to say about those three issues. We can see how pale pure science is when compared with moral urgency and hermeneutic creativity.

Next I have to face the ultimate anthropological question about science: how do other cultures treat science? The most basic instinct of the anthropologist is to ask, "What happens in other cultures?" If many different peoples behave or believe in a similar way, that produces a cross-cultural generalization, a sort of descriptive law of human nature. But when another culture has a unique way of responding to a given problem, then we have to discard our cross-cultural laws and consider only what this information tells us about one particular culture. The cross-cultural laws give us knowledge that is broad but not particularly deep; the unique cases lead to insights that are deep but not very broad. Some of the lessons of anthropology are broad, and some are deep, but most fall into a murky realm that is not as broad as universal laws of human nature and not so deep as to be utterly unique to only one culture. Such is the curse of cultural anthropology.

Until now I have postponed the question of science in other cultures so that I could do a solid job with the one culture I know best. But I realize that the question deserves some thought. To take but one problem, remember that the European scientific research ethos came from Europe, in which case we might well ask how that ethos has since evolved in Europe and how it interacts with the different European national cultures.

In a book on medicine and culture, Lynn Payer reminds the reader that modern medicine is believed to be an objective science that transcends the idiosyncrasies of the various Western cultures. But then she shows how thoroughly medicine is situated in national tradition. French medicine celebrates and reflects the French people's love of abstract rationalism; German medicine is strongly metaphysical, even including homeopathy and hydrotherapy within mainstream practice; British medicine emphasizes that a person builds character by stoically enduring discomfort. Diagnosis and therapy, including both prescriptions and surgery, depend to some extent on the values and meanings of each national culture.[17] My hunch is that science changes just as much from culture to culture as does medicine.

Do other cultures have other ways of conjuring science? I cannot answer that question here, but I can suggest a sequence of three queries that will lead to an answer for a given culture. First, how does this culture balance respect for science with understanding of science? Respect without understanding, also known as science in an Old Testament style, is a necessary condition for the conjuring of science. But if the status of science is somewhat less than that of a mysterious religion having a plenary authority, there is less temptation to hijack that kind of authority for causes that have little or nothing to do with science.

Second, which extrinsic meanings and values might be invested in science? Which might benefit from the conjuring of science? These questions ought to narrow the range of phenomena to look for, if the supposed plenary authority of science lends itself more readily to some cultural meanings than to others. I must admit, however, that the American experience of conjuring science is hopelessly promiscuous. There is no apparent restriction to the variety of cultural meanings that can become cloaked in scientific respectability, as evidenced by the five episodes in this book. God help us if this is also true of many other cultures.

Third, what are the popular symbols of science in this culture, and how can they be transferred from science to nonscientific meanings? Meanings need symbols. Thus, we can ideally find symbols by first finding the meanings that generate them, or we can find meanings by working back from the symbols we see. At any rate, culture is, by the definition of interpretive anthropology, a system of meanings and symbols, and a unique culture is a unique configuration of meanings and symbols. It must have a repertoire of popular symbols of science if the authority of science is to be attributed to extrascientific meanings.

Those are the loose ends I leave behind me. Instead of tying them up neatly, I invite you to expand my views or amend them or refute them by testing my ideas against other episodes or other cultures.

■ ■ ■

What, then, should we think of science? Actually, I do not know much about the metaphysical value of scientific knowledge. As a cultural anthropologist, I am agnostic in most disputes that set one scientific argument against another. I am also the guy who earned a *D* in freshman biology thirty years ago and an *F* in computer science two years after that. More often than not, I lack the wisdom and the credentials to pass judgment on competing scientific claims. Instead, my modest contribution is to ask about the hermeneutics of science, about how we borrow the authority of science to corroborate our own meanings and values within the messy realm of democratic science.

I conclude that science is culturally hollow. This institution carelessly allows its meanings and values to be eviscerated when it permits mischiefmakers to hijack its symbols for the benefit of other values and meanings. This is not to say that science lacks intrinsic values, morality, or ethics. At the very least, science cherishes rationalism, secularism, naturalism, and science for the sake of science, plus numerous secondary values derived from those four. But then scientists foolishly allow anyone to steal the intangible benefits of their work, namely, the institutional authority of science.

If a millionaire amassed a great collection of cash but then left the mansion unguarded and the front door open, would we not say that this is obviously foolish? If scientists amass enormous credibility by adhering to good values and rigorous methods but then invite anyone to help himself or herself to that credibility, should we not say that this, too, is obviously foolish? To compound this folly, the language of science, as described in Geertz's Observation, makes scientists blind to the hermeneutic larceny going on around them.

And what about the rest of us? We are not the kind of people who burglarize science for its plenary authority, are we? We do not commit the criminal deed. But what if we are consumers of conjured science? Science is going to touch our lives; that is unavoidable. But when we permit an ersatz substitute, assembled by conjurers from smoke and mirrors, to shape the values in our hearts and mark the paths of our actions, then we are asking for trouble. Is this not like buying contraband computer chips or counterfeits of name-brand watches or knockoffs of designer clothes? The price is right, but after a while their inferior quality becomes apparent as they break down or fall apart.

I hope the same is true about the consumption of conjured science: that its folly will become apparent before long. But I fear this will not happen. I fear that for many people conjured science is a satisfactory stand-in for science because science too often ignores or suppresses the cultural meanings we need to make sense of our lives, whereas conjured science, by definition, affirms such meanings.

NOTES

■ ■ ■

1. Science in an Old Testament Style

1. Downey 1986:398, 1988:36; Keeney 1989:1203; LaFollette 1990:100–101; McElheny 1985:277; Nelkin 1987:71, 78; Rosenberg 1966:136; Whalen 1981:16.

2. LaFollette 1990:156; McElheny 1985:277; Whalen 1981:16.

2. American Visions of Nature and Science

1. Bruce 1987:68; see also Conser 1993:4.

2. Burnham 1987:23; Hollinger 1989; Keeney 1989:1206; Marsden 1980:111–112, 1989; McIver 1989:12–25; Sandeen 1967:73, 1970:169; Webb 1983; Toumey 1991.

3. Grave 1960:112–114; McIver 1989:15–19; Olson 1975: chap. 1; Webb 1983, 1994:16.

4. Hughes 1983:112; McIver 1989:15–25; Webb 1983.

5. Bruce 1987:34.

6. Marsden 1980:111–112; McIver 1989:12; Sandeen 1967:73, 1970:169.

7. Marsden 1980:110; see also Webb 1994:16.

8. Conser 1993:9.

9. Bruce 1987:5.

10. Meier 1957; Marx 1987; Harrison 1992.

11. Meier 1957:623.

12. Marx 1987:37–38.

13. Meier 1957; Daniels 1967; Marx 1987.

14. Cf. Downey 1986:392–394.

15. Meier 1957:625.

16. Ferguson 1979:3; 14–15; Meier 1957:627.

17. Downey 1986:392.

18. Meier 1957:626.

19. Ferguson 1979:4.

20. Cf. Daniels 1967:1699–1700; Keeney 1989:1205; Price 1968:8–9; Massey 1989:915.

21. Tocqueville 1899:518, 527.

22. Tocqueville 1899:523.

23. Tocqueville 1899:523.

24. Tocqueville 1899:524.

25. Tocqueville 1899:519.

26. Reingold 1987:137.

27. Bruce 1987:7–13; Reingold 1987.

28. Daniels 1967:1700.

29. Cf. Rosenberg 1966:159; Price 1968:14.

30. Bruce 1987:8.

31. Daniels 1967:1702–1703.

32. Conser 1993:138.

33. Conser 1993:138.

34. Burnham 1987:173; 226; Rosenberg 1966:159; Keeney 1989:1208.

35. Burnham 1987; LaFollette 1990.

36. Burnham 1987:5, 248. Cf. Basalla 1976 for an analysis similar to Burnham's and LaFollette's; see also Bruce 1987:118.

37. Grabiner and Miller 1974:836.

38. Cf. Ashby 1960:1166; Burnham 1987:205; Raman 1975:9–10; Rosenberg 1966; Rowland 1993:1571; Whitley 1985:5.

3. Democratic Culture and the Moral Autonomy of Science

1. Reingold 1978:61, 1979:19; Daniels 1967:1699, 1704.

2. Bruce 1987:225.

3. Hollinger 1983.

4. Merton 1973a, 1973b; Hollinger 1983.

5. Hollinger 1983.

6. Shapin 1993:839.

7. Ben-David 1984: 169–176.

8. Piel 1986:1059.

9. Bush 1960:12, 33.

10. Piel 1986:1059.

11. Crease and Samios 1991; Daniels 1967:1704; Guston and Keniston 1994; Piel 1986:1059; Roush 1992:57.

12. Daniels 1967:1704–1705.

13. Reingold 1979:19.

14. Barnes 1989; Rainie and Cohen 1991; Roush 1992.

15. Cohen 1993; Garment 1991:163–165.

16. Roush 1992:57–58; Garment 1991:164.

17. Garment 1991:165–166.

18. Garment 1991:164.

19. Garment 1991:167–168.

20. Garment 1991:9.

21. Shilts 1988:95.

22. Shilts 1988:93.

23. Shilts 1988:614–615.

24. Anderson 1993.

25. Roush 1992:62.

26. See Guston and Keniston 1994.

27. LaFollette 1990.9.

28. Dewey 1966:223; Burnham 1987:32; Keeney 1989:1209; Holton 1960:1188.

29. Lincoln 1991:74.

30. Price 1968:24–25; Tobey 1971:13. Cf. Smith 1991.

31. Ezrahi 1990:67–96.

32. Shortland 1988:311–313.

33. Dewey 1931:328, 1966:225.

34. Dewey 1931:329.

35. Dewey 1966:230.

36. Dewey 1931:330.

37. Popper 1950:3–6, 407–411.

38. Bell 1960.

39. Popper 1950:11.

40. Miller 1987a:34, 1983, 1987b.

41. Miller 1983:29, 1987b:26,

42. Miller 1987b:28. John Durant's research in the United Kingdom finds the same results there (Culliton 1989:600).

43. Nelkin 1987:6.

44. Nelkin 1987:7. Cf. Raman 1975:14.

45. Nelkin 1987:7.

46. Burnham 1987.

47. Mazur 1981.

48. Shortland 1988:313.

49. Cf. Culliton 1989:600; Miller 1987a:30; Langenberg 1991:361.

50. Burnham 1987:179; Culliton 1989:600; Miller 1987a:35, 1987b:30.

51. *Science,* March 11, 1988, 239:1237; Pfeiffenberger, Zolandz, and Jones 1991:36.

52. *Science,* February 10, 1989, 243:229.

53. *Science,* July 3, 1992, 257:26; Stevenson 1992:70–71; Stevenson, Chen, and Lee 1993.

54. Pfeiffenberger, Zolandz, and Jones 1991:36.

55. *Science,* March 11, 1988, 239:1237; Pfeiffenberger, Zolandz, and Jones 1991:36; Stevenson 1992:70–71.

56. *Science,* September 30, 1988, 241:1751; see also *Chronicle of Higher Education,* November 8, 1989; A37.

57. *Science,* March 11, 1988, 239:1237.

58. Rutherford 1985:207–209.

59. Mead and Metraux 1957:384.

60. Beardslee and O'Dowd 1961:997.

61. Beardslee and O'Dowd 1961:997.

62. Shallis and Hills 1975.

63. Ferris 1993:18.

64. Larson 1985:4–5.

65. Cf. Langenberg 1991:361.

66. Larson 1985:170–171.

67. Sclove 1994.

68. Sclove 1995b.

69. Winner 1992:356–358.

70. Winner 1992:358.

71. Sclove 1995a.

72. Winner 1986.

73. Winner 1994:72.

74. Winner 1992:354.

4. Scientific Symbols and Cultural Meanings

1. Geertz 1973:91.

2. Peacock 1975:1–2.

3. Geertz 1983:118.

4. Geertz 1983:21.

5. Downey 1986.

6. Downey 1986:408.

7. Downey 1986:409.

8. Baudrillard 1983b, 1988.

9. Baudrillard 1988:170.

10. Cf. Geertz's essay on ideology, 1973:193–233.

11. Baudrillard 1983b:2–12.

12. Baudrillard 1983b:4–6.

13. Baudrillard 1983a:95, 100, 103.

14. Baudrillard 1988:209.

15. Baudrillard 1988:209.

16. Baudrillard 1983b:3.

17. Mander 1978:261.

18. Mander 1978:250.

19. Mander 1978:252.
20. Mander 1978:255.
21. Mander 1978:266–275.
22. Mander 1978:269.
23. Mander 1978:308.
24. Mander 1978:302–310.
25. Mander 1978:323–328.
26. Rosenberg 1966.
27. Rosenberg 1966.
28. Rosenberg 1966:143.
29. Rosenberg 1966:136.

5. Soul-Snatching

1. Sapolsky 1968:428.
2. Hastreiter 1983:486; Martin 1991:2–3; Paul 1961:1.
3. Shaw 1954:233.
4. Shaw 1954:235.
5. Martin 1991:4; Paul 1961:2.
6. Shaw 1954:237–238.
7. Sapolsky 1968:428.
8. Frazier 1980; Kirscht 1961:16–26; Mausner and Mausner 1955:38; Paul 1959:19; Plaut 1959:214, 222; Simmel and Ast 1962:1270–1272.
9. Mausner and Mausner 1955.
10. Paul 1959:20; Lear 1963:77.
11. Paul 1961:2.
12. Mausner and Mausner 1955:36.
13. Shaw 1954.
14. Shaw 1954:233
15. Lear 1963:77.
16. Green 1961:16–17, 24.
17. Mausner and Mausner 1955; Paul 1959, 1961; Plaut 1959, 1960; Gamson 1961; Green 1961; Simmel and Ast 1962; Sapolsky 1968. See also Martin's critique of this thinking: Martin 1988:335–336; 1989.
18. Mausner and Mausner 1955:39.
19. Consumers Union 1978a:394; Margolis and Cohen 1985:115.
20. Margolis and Cohen 1985:115–16.
21. Consumers Union 1978a, 1978b.
22. Hileman 1988:36–37.
23. Smith 1988:454.
24. Smith 1988:455, 456, 457, 459.
25. Martin 1988:356.
26. Martin 1988:347.

27. Martin 1989.

28. Martin 1991:8, 11.

29. Martin 1988:355.

30. Martin 1988:335, 1989:69.

31. Martin 1991:56 ff.

32. *Science,* January 19, 1990, 247:276–277; *Newsweek,* February 5, 1990: 60–61.

33. National Research Council 1993:1–2.

34. White 1956.

35. Jensen 1971.

36. Jensen 1971:37.

37. Jensen 1971:38.

38. Mausner and Mausner 1955; Green 1961.

39. Sapolsky 1968:430.

40. Kirscht 1961:23; Gamson 1961:5–6.

41. Paul 1959:20; Green 1961:16–17; Lear 1963:77.

42. Green 1961:16–17; see also Paul 1959:20; Lear 1964:92.

43. Kilpatrick 1990.

44. Kilpatrick 1990.

45. Green 1961:14.

46. Green 1961:14.

47. Mausner and Mausner 1955:36–38.

48. Plaut 1959:216.

49. Lear 1963, 1964.

50. Rodale 1961:878.

51. Paul 1959:19; Mausner and Mausner 1955:36.

52. Martin 1988:331; see also Margolis and Cohen 1985:116; Mausner and Mausner 1955:38; Sapolsky 1968:431; Mueller 1968:1876–1879; Davis 1959:482.

53. Lear 1963, 1964; Hileman 1988; Smith 1988. Cf. Kirscht and Knutson 1961:42.

54. Paul 1959:20, 1961:5.

55. Paul 1959:20.

56. Paul 1959:20.

57. Martin 1988, 1991:56–91. Note also that Martin has added some very thoughtful comments about his stance on fluoridation, and its more general implications for the sociology of scientific knowledge, in Scott, Richards, and Martin 1990.

58. Green 1961.

6. *Plague*

1. Fox 1988.

2. Fox 1988; see also Fee and Fox 1992.
3. Shilts 1988:149–50.
4. Altman 1986:33; Oppenheimer 1988:271–275; Shilts 1988:156.
5. Combie 1990:18–19.
6. Herek and Glunt 1988:889; Altman 1986:1–2; Brandt 1988:379.
7. Burnham 1987:75–76.
8. Shilts 1988:300, 321, 586.
9. Altman 1986:180.
10. Shilts 1988:301, 419.
11. Shilts 1988.
12. Duesberg 1981, 1989, 1991; Curtis 1992.
13. EIR 1983:1.
14. EIR 1983; LaRouche 1987; King 1989.
15. LaRouche 1987:4, 185, 325–326.
16. EIR 1983:161–240.
17. EIR 1983:178; 184, 161–240.
18. King 1989:139.
19. King 1989:156.
20. King 1989:143–144.
21. King 1989:139.
22. King 1989:140–141; 275–278.
23. EIR 1983:161.
24. LaRouche 1987:vii.
25. LaRouche 1987:171.
26. LaRouche 1987:321.
27. EIR 1988:4
28. King 1989:139–141.
29. EIR 1988:3.
30. EIR 1988:4, 95, 156, 175.
31. EIR 1988:3, 17.
32. EIR 1988:4, 25; LaRouche 1987:324; *Los Angeles Times,* February 6, 1988.
33. Seale 1984, 1986, 1987a, 1987b, 1988.
34. Krieger and Lashof 1988:411.
35. *Science,* October 17, 1986, 234:277.
36. Krieger and Lashof 1988; King 1989:140.
37. *L.A. Times,* June 24, 1986.
38. *L.A. Times,* August 3, 1986.
39. *L.A. Times,* August 12, 1986.
40. *L.A. Times,* August 9, 1986.
41. *L.A. Times,* August 12, 1986.
42. NDPC 1986:13.

43. *New Statesman,* November 7, 1986:7.
44. *L.A. Times,* August 3, 1986.
45. NDPC 1986:2.
46. *L.A. Times,* August 3, 1986.
47. NDPC 1986:2; *L.A. Times,* October 4, 1986.
48. *New Statesman,* November 7, 1986:7–8.
49. EIR 1983.
50. NDPC 1986.
51. *L.A. Times,* August 3, 1986.
52. *L.A. Times,* September 18, 1986.
53. *Science,* October 17, 1986, 234:278; *L.A. Times,* August 9, 1986.
54. *L.A. Times,* July 13, 1986; *L.A. Times,* October 30, 1986.
55. NDPC 1986:1.
56. *L.A. Times,* August 3, 1986.
57. *Science,* October 17, 1986, 234:278.
58. Rundall and Phillips 1990:5.
59. King 1989:142–43.
60. King 1989:143.
61. Downey 1988:27.
62. Mulkay 1979:114.

7. Hope

1. Taubes 1993, Rousseau 1992; Huizenga 1992.
2. Pool 1989:423; Taubes 1993:214.
3. NOVA 1990:1.
4. Heylin 1990:25.
5. Heylin 1990:25.
6. *Chronicle of Higher Education,* May 3, 1989:A6.
7. *Wall Street Journal,* March 24, 1989:A1. Peat 1989:13.
8. *Chronicle of Higher Education,* May 3, 1989:A6.
9. Peat 1989:102–103; see also Crawford 1989:522; Huizenga 1992:50–51; Taubes 1993:251.
10. NOVA 1990:8.
11. NOVA 1990:7.
12. Taubes 1993:115.
13. *Newsweek,* May 1, 1989:66.
14. *Chronicle of Higher Education,* May 10, 1989:A4; see also, *Nature,* May 4, 1989, 339:4.
15. *Science,* July 21, 1989, 245:256.
16. Taubes 1993:112.
17. Taubes 1993:175.
18. *Wall Street Journal,* April 12, 1989:A14.

19. Huizenga 1992:174.

20. *Business Week,* August 24, 1992:77; October 26, 1992:120; November 9, 1992:109.

21. NOVA 1990:7; see also Huizenga 1992:44.

22. *Science,* May 12, 1989, 244:647.

23. Taubes 1993:293.

24. Huizenga 1992:173.

25. Huizenga 1992:173.

26. Peat 1989:76.

27. *Newsweek,* May 15, 1989:65.

28. *Chronicle of Higher Education,* May 24, 1989:A8; Heylin 1990:25.

29. *Chronicle of Higher Education,* May 24, 1989:A10.

30. *Chronicle of Higher Education,* April 19, 1989:A10.

31. Bockris 1991:51.

32. Peat 1989:109.

33. NOVA 1990:6.

34. Huizenga 1992:166; NOVA 1990:6–7.

35. Taubes 1993:285.

36. Bockris 1991:51; *Chronicle of Higher Education,* April 11, 1990:A8.

37. *Chronicle of Higher Education,* August 14, 1991:A6.

38. Goodstein 1994:530.

39. Close 1993:83.

40. Port 1992; *Science,* April 3, 1992, 254:28; *Business Week,* August 24, 1992:77.

41. Taubes 1993:428; Goodstein 1994:537; Storms 1994.

42. *Chronicle of Higher Education,* December 15, 1993:A18.

43. *Science,* December 18, 1992, 258:1879.

44. Close 1991; Huizenga 1992; Taubes 1993; Mallove 1991.

45. Peat 1989.

46. *Science,* February 4, 1994, 263:607.

47. Storms 1994.

48. Storms 1994:29.

49. Lewenstein 1995:127.

50. Goodstein 1994:527.

8. Anarchy

1. 370 US 421; 374 US 203.

2. 367 US 495.

3. 380 US 193.

4. Whitehead and Conlan 1978; LaHaye 1980; McGraw 1976; ProFamily Forum 1980.

5. 374 US 225.

6. Rafferty 1969:11, 42, 71–72.

7. Nelkin 1982:100–101.

8. McGraw 1976:8–9.

9. *New York Times,* April 12, 1978, December 14, 1978, May 19, 1979; *Science,* June 1, 1979, 204:925.

10. Whitehead and Conlan 1978.

11. For a more conventional account of the same legal history, see Hammond 1984.

12. *New Humanist,* May–June 1933; *The Humanist,* September–October 1973; Whitehead and Conlan 1978:30–31, 44.

13. Whitehead and Conlan 1978:45; 19.

14. LaHaye 1980:9, 26.

15. LaHaye 1980:85.

16. Hadden and Swann 1981:86.

17. *News and Observer* (Raleigh, N.C.), May 12, 1985.

18. *Newsweek,* July 6, 1981:48.

19. *Bible-Science Newsletter,* May 1984: 7 (insert).

20. Bolles.

21. *Charlotte Observer,* June 13, 1980.

22. ProFamily Forum 1980.

23. *Creation-Science Report,* December 1978.

24. *New Humanist,* May–June 1933.

25. *The Humanist,* September–October 1973.

26. Kurtz 1985:330, 332.

27. Gale 1987:1607–1608.

28. LaHaye 1980:179; *N.Y. Times,* August 26, 1973.

29. Abbagnano 1967:71; Giustiniani 1985:192–193.

30. O'Brien 1979:1734.

31. Kurtz 1989.

32. *N.Y. Times,* December 17, 1972.

33. Morris 1972:271.

34. Morris and Gish 1976:315.

35. *N.Y. Times,* December 14, 1978.

36. Morris 1984:328.

37. Wysong 1976:6.

38. Mayr 1978:53.

39. Newell 1974.

40. Pollitzer 1980:329–330.

41. Bryan 1922:243.

42. *Time,* March 16, 1981:82.

43. Morris 1963:93.

44. Morris 1974:74–75.

45. Morris 1984:223.
46. Morris and Gish 1976:172.
47. Morris 1982, 1983, 1987, 1984:352.
48. McIver 1989:294–302; Harrison 1990.
49. *Science,* March 20, 1981, 211:1331–1332; *Science,* June 1, 1979, 204:925.
50. *Bible-Science Newsletter,* March 1975.
51. Morris, Gish, and Hillestad 1974:27.
52. *Acts and Facts* (monthly newsletter of ICR), July 1983.
53. *Creation Science Prayer News,* August 1985.
54. OTGH 1981.
55. Chick 1976.
56. Chick 1972.

9. Evil

1. Sontag 1966:216.
2. Sontag 1966:223.
3. Brustein 1958:296.
4. Prawer 1980:85.
5. Murray 1972:109.
6. Murray 1972:292.
7. Murray 1972:293.
8. Murray 1972:111.
9. Prawer 1980:85.
10. Murray 1972:294.
11. Glut 1978:138.
12. Glut 1978:146.
13. Glut 1978:148, 157.
14. Goldsmith 1981:16.
15. Friedman 1984:132.
16. Goldsmith 1981:16–17; Friedman 1984:131.
17. Shelley 1964:xi–xii.
18. Shelley 1964:33.
19. Shelley 1964:40.
20. Cf. Levine 1979:10; Lawler 1988:255.
21. Friedman 1964:132.
22. Shelley 1964:47.
23. Shelley 1964:240.
24. Nitchie 1953:224; LaValley 1979:249.
25. LaValley 1979:247.
26. Nitchie 1953:221.
27. Huss and Ross 1972.

28. Mank 1981:13.
29. Mank 1981:17; LaValley 1979:259.
30. Mank 1981:3.
31. Mank 1981:1.
32. Mank 1981:46.
33. Mank 1981:93.
34. Pirie 1973:72; see also Glut 1973:189, 195.
35. Pirie 1973:70.
36. Pirie 1973:73, 74.
37. Pirie 1973:79.
38. Cf. LaValley 1979:277.
39. Stevenson 1984:678.
40. Stevenson 1984:679.
41. Stevenson 1984:684.
42. Glut 1978:75; Wilstach 1983:159.
43. Prawer 1980:106; Saposnik 1983:115.
44. Prawer 1980:86.
45. Clarens 1967:41.
46. Prawer 1980:92–93; Clarens 1967:83.
47. Prawer 1980:105.
48. Glut 1978:103.

10. A Manual for Conjurers

1. Rosenberg 1966.
2. Burnham 1987; LaFollette 1990.
3. Burnham 1987:232.
4. Larson 1985.
5. Downey 1988:27.
6. *The Imaginary Invalid,* 3.14.
7. Crossen 1994:21–22.
8. Crossen 1994:161–166; *Chronicle of Higher Education,* December 14, 1994:A26–31.
9. Scalia 1987, 55 LW 4872.
10. Peter Sandman, David Sachsman, and Michael Greenberg, cited in Cohn 1990:18.
11. Paul 1959:20, 1961.
12. Taubes 1995.
13. Mazur 1981.
14. *Science,* April 22, 1994, 264:500–501.
15. *Newsweek,* May 22, 1995:47.
16. Geertz 1973:231; see also 111.
17. Payer 1988.

BIBLIOGRAPHY

■ ■ ■

Abbagnano, Nicola. 1967. "Humanism." *Encyclopedia of Philosophy,* ed. P. Edwards, 4:69–72. New York: Macmillan.

Altman, Dennis. 1986. *AIDS in the Mind of America.* Garden City, N.Y.: Doubleday.

Anderson, Christopher. 1993. "Bromley's Last Stand." *Science,* January 1, 259:20–21.

Ashby, Eric. 1960. "Dons or Crooners?" *Science,* April 22, 131:1165–1170.

Barnes, Fred. 1989. "Bad Cop." *New Republic,* October 23:10–12.

Basalla, George. 1976. "Pop Science: The Depiction of Science in Popular Culture." In *Science and Its Public,* ed. G. Holton and W. A. Blanpied, 261–278. Boston: Reidel.

Baudrillard, Jean. 1983a. *In the Shadow of the Silent Majorities...or The End of the Social, and Other Essays.* New York: Semiotexte.

———. 1983b. *Simulations.* New York: Semiotexte.

———. 1988. *Selected Writings.* ed. M. Poster. Stanford, Calif.: Stanford University Press.

Beardslee, David C., and Donald D. O'Dowd. 1961. "The College-Student Image of the Scientist." *Science,* March 31, 133:997–1001.

Bell, Daniel. 1960. *The End of Ideology.* Glencoe, Ill.: Free Press.

Ben-David, Joseph. 1984 [1971]. *The Scientist's Role in Society.* Chicago: University of Chicago Press.

Bockris, John. 1991. "Cold Fusion II: The Story Continues." *New Scientist,* January 19:50–53.

Bolles, T. H. N.d. "Humanism: America's Greatest Enemy." White Bear Lake, Minn.: Victory. Tract.

Brandt, Allen M. 1988. "The Syphilis Epidemic and Its Relation to AIDS." *Science,* January 22, 239:375–380.

Bruce, Robert V. 1987. *The Launching of American Science, 1846–1876.* New York: Knopf.

Brustein, Robert. 1958. "Reflections on Horror Movies." *Partisan Review,* Spring, 25(2):288–296.

Bryan, William Jennings. 1922. "William Jennings Bryan on Evolution." *Science,* March 3, 15:242–243.

Burnham, John C. 1987. *How Superstition Won and Science Lost: Popularizing Science and Health in the United States.* New Brunswick, N.J.: Rutgers University Press.

Bush, Vannevar. 1960 [1945]. *Science, the Endless Frontier: A Report to the President on a Program for Postwar Scientific Research.* Washington, D.C.: National Science Foundation.

Chick, Jack T. 1972. "Big Daddy?" Comic-book tract. Chino, Calif.: Chick Publications.

———. 1976 "Primal Man?" Comic-book tract. Chino, Calif.: Chick Publications.

Clarens, Carlos. 1967. *An Illustrated History of the Horror Film.* New York: Capricorn.

Close, Frank. 1991. *Too Hot to Handle: The Race for Cold Fusion.* Princeton: Princeton University Press.

———. 1993. "From Farce to Fiasco." *American Scientist,* January–February 1993:83–84.

Cohen, I. Bernard. 1963. "Science in America: The Nineteenth Century." In *Paths of American Thought,* ed. A. M. Schlesinger Jr. and M. White, 167–189. Boston: Houghton Mifflin.

Cohen, John. 1993. "HHS: Gallo Guilty of Misconduct." *Science,* January 8, 259:168–170.

Cohn, Victor. 1990. *Reporting Risk.* Washington, D.C.: Media Institute.

Combie, S.C. 1990. "AIDS in Cultural, Historic, and Epidemiologic Context." In *Culture and AIDS,* ed. D. A. Feldman, 9–27. New York: Praeger.

Conser, Walter H. Jr. 1993. *God and the Natural World: Religion and Science in Antebellum America.* Columbia: University of South Carolina Press.

Consumers Union. 1978a. "Fluoridation: The Cancer Scare." *Consumer Reports,* July:392–396.

———. 1978b. "Six Ways to Mislead the Public." *Consumer Reports,* August: 480–482.

Crawford, Mark. 1989. "Utah Looks to Congress for Cold Fusion Cash." *Science,* May 5, 244:522–523.

Crease, Robert P., and Nicholas P. Samios. 1991. "Managing the Unmanageable." *Atlantic Monthly,* January:80–88.

Crossen, Cynthia. 1994. *Tainted Truth.* New York: Simon and Schuster.

Culliton, Barbara J. 1989. "The Dismal State of Scientific Literacy." *Science,* February 3, 243:600.

Curtis, Tom. 1992. "The Origin of AIDS." *Rolling Stone,* March 19:54 ff.

Daniels, George H. 1967. "The Pure-Science Ideal and Democratic Culture." *Science,* June 30, 156:1699–1705.

Davis, Morris. 1959. "Community Attitudes Towards Fluoridation." *Public Opinion Quarterly* 13:474–482.

Dewey, John. 1931. *Philosophy and Civilization.* New York: Putnam's Sons.

———. 1966 [1916]. *Democracy and Education.* New York: Free Press.

Downey, Gary. 1986. "Risk in Culture: The American Conflict over Nuclear Power." *Cultural Anthropology* 1(4):388–412.

———. 1988. "Structure and Practice in the Cultural Identities of Scientists: Negotiating Nuclear Waste in New Mexico." *Anthropological Quarterly* 61(1):26–38.

Duesberg, Peter H. 1987. "Retroviruses as Carcinogens and Pathogens: Expectations and Reality." *Cancer Research* 47, March 1:1199–1220.

———. 1989. "Human Immunodeficiency Virus and Acquired Immune Deficiency Syndrome: Correlation but Not Causation." *Proceedings of the National Academy of Sciences* 86, February: 755–764.

———. 1991. "AIDS Epidemiology: Inconsistencies with Human Immunodeficiency Virus and with Infectious Disease." *Proceedings of the National Academy of Sciences* 88, February:1575–1579.

Durkheim, Emile. 1965 [1912]. *The Elementary Forms of the Religious Life.* New York: Free Press.

Durkheim, Emile and Marcel Mauss. 1963 [1903]. *Primitive Classification.* Chicago: University of Chicago Press.

EIR (editors of *Executive Intelligence Review*). 1983. *LaRouche: Will This Man Be President?* New York: New Benjamin Franklin House.

———. 1988. *AIDS Global Showdown: Mankind's Total Victory or Total Defeat.* Washington, D.C.: Executive Intelligence Review.

Ezrahi, Yaron 1990. *The Descent of Icarus: Science and the Transformation of Democracy.* Cambridge: Cambridge University Press.

Fee, Elizabeth, and Daniel M. Fox. 1992. "The Contemporary Historiography of AIDS." In *AIDS: The Making of a Chronic Disease,* ed. E. Fee and D. M. Fox, 1–19. Berkeley and Los Angeles: University of Calif. Press.

Ferguson, Eugene S. 1979. "The American-ness of American Technology." *Technology and Culture* 20(1):3–24.

Ferris, Timothy. 1993. "The Case Against Science." *New York Review of Books,* May 13:17–19.

Fox, Daniel M. 1988. "AIDS and the American Health Polity: The History and Prospects of a Crisis of Authority." In *AIDS: The Burden of History,* ed. E. Fee and D. M. Fox, 316–343. Berkeley and Los Angeles: University of Calif. Press.

Frazier, P. Jean. 1980. "Fluoridation: A Review of Social Research." *Journal of Public Health Dentistry* 40(3):214–233.

Friedman, Lester D. 1984. "'Canyons of Nightmare': The Jewish Horror Film." In *Planks of Reason: Essays on the Horror Film*, ed. B. K. Grant, 126–152. Metuchen, N.J.: Scarecrow.

Gale. 1987. *Encyclopedia of Associations 1988*. 22nd ed. Vol. 1, part 2. Detroit: Gale Publishing.

Gamson, William A. 1961. "Social Science Aspects of Fluoridation." *Health Education Journal*, September:1–11.

Garment, Suzanne. 1991. *Scandal: The Culture of Mistrust in American Politics*. New York: Random House.

Geertz, Clifford. 1973. *The Interpretation of Cultures*. New York: Basic Books.

———. 1983. *Local Knowledge*. New York: Basic Books.

Giustiniani, Vito R. 1985. "Homo, Humanus, and the Meanings of 'Humanism.'" *Journal of the History of Ideas* 46(2):167–195.

Glut, D. F. 1973. *The Frankenstein Legend*. Metuchen, N.J.: Scarecrow.

———. 1978. *Classic Movie Monsters*. Metuchen, N.J.: Scarecrow.

Goldsmith, Arnold L. 1981. *The Golem Remembered, 1909–1980*. Detroit: Wayne State University Press.

Goodstein, David. 1994. "Pariah Science." *American Scholar* 63:527–541.

Gould, Stephen Jay. 1981. "Evolution as Fact and Theory." *Discover*, May:34–37.

Grabiner, Judith V., and Peter D. Miller. 1974. "Effects of the Scopes Trial." *Science*, September 6, 185:832–837.

Grave, S. A. 1960. *The Scottish Common Sense Philosophy*. Westport, Conn.: Greenwood.

Green, Arnold L. 1961. "The Ideology of the Anti-Fluoridation Leaders." *Journal of Social Issues* 17(4):13–25.

Guston, David H., and Kenneth Keniston. 1994. "Updating the Social Contract for Science." *Technology Review*, November-December:61–68.

Hadden, Jeffrey K., and Charles E. Swann. 1981. *Prime Time Preachers*. Reading, Mass.: Addison-Wesley.

Hammond, Phillip E. 1984. "The Courts and Secular Humanism." *Society*, May–June:11–16.

Harrison, Lester H. 1990. "Creationism as a Moral Critique." Paper presented at the symposium "Science, Knowledge, and Technology" at the Annual Meeting of the Southwestern Social Science Association, Fort Worth, Texas, March.

———. 1992. "The Fate of Science in America." Paper presented at the symposium "Science, Knowledge, and Technology" at the Annual Meeting of Southwestern Social Science Association, Austin, Texas, March.

Hastreiter, Richard J. 1983. "Fluoridation Conflict: A History and Conceptual Synthesis." *Journal of the American Dental Association*, 106:486–490.

Herek, Gregory M., and Eric K. Glunt. 1988. "An Epidemic of Stigma." *American Psychologist* 43:886–891.

Heylin, Michael. 1990. "Sociology of Cold Fusion Examined." *Chemical and Engineering News,* March 19:24–25.

Hileman, Bette. 1988. "Fluoridation of Water." *Chemical and Engineering News,* August 1:26–42.

Hollinger, David A. 1983. "The Defense of Democracy and Robert K. Merton's Formulation of the Scientific Ethos." *Knowledge and Society* 4:1–15.

———. 1989. "Justification by Verification: The Scientific Challenge to the Moral Authority of Christianity in Modern America." In *Religion and Twentieth-Century American Intellectual Life,* ed. M. J. Lacy, 116–135. Cambridge: Cambridge University Press.

Holton, Gerald. 1960. "Modern Science and the Intellectual Tradition." *Science,* April 22, 131:1187–1193.

Hughes, H. Stuart. 1983. "Social Theory in a New Context." In *The Muses Flee Hitler,* ed. J. C. Jackman and C. M. Border, 111–120. Washington, D.C.: Smithsonian Institution Press.

Huizenga, John R. 1992. *Cold Fusion: The Scientific Fiasco of the Century.* Rochester, New York: University of Rochester Press.

Huss, Roy, and T. J. Ross. 1972. *Focus on the Horror Film.* Englewood Cliffs, N.J.: Prentice-Hall.

Jensen, Paul. 1971. "The Return of Dr. Caligari." *Film Comment,* Winter, 7(4):36–45.

Keeney, Elizabeth Barnaby. 1989. "Science." In *Handbook of American Popular Culture,* ed. M. T. Inge, 3:1203–1228. 2d. ed. rev. Westport, Conn: Greenwood.

King, Dennis. 1989. *Lyndon LaRouche and the New American Fascism.* New York: Doubleday.

Kilpatrick, James J. 1990. "Fluoridation Fiats Trounce Personal Freedom." *News and Observer* (Raleigh, N.C.), February 9, op.-ed. col.

Kirscht, John P. 1961. "Attitude Research on the Fluoridation Controversy." *Health Education Monographs* 10:16–28.

Kirscht, John P., and Andie L. Knutson. 1961. "Science and Fluoridation: An Attitude Survey." *Journal of Social Issues* 17(4):37–44.

Krieger, Nancy, and Joyce Lashof. 1988. "AIDS, Policy Analysis, and the Electorate: The Role of Schools of Public Health." *American Journal of Public Health,* April, 78:411–15.

Kurtz, Paul. 1985. "Humanism." *Encyclopedia of Unbelief,* ed. G. Stein, 1:328–333. Buffalo, N.Y.: Prometheus.

———. 1989. "The New Age in Perspective." *Skeptical Inquirer* 13:365–367.

LaHaye, Tim. 1980. *The Battle for the Mind.* Old Tappan, N.J.: Fleming H. Revell.

LaFollette, Marcel. 1990. *Making Science Our Own: Public Images of Science, 1910–1955.* Chicago: University of Chicago Press.

Langenberg, Donald N. 1991. "Science, Slogans, and Civic Duty." *Science,* April 19, 252:361–363.

LaRouche, Lyndon H. Jr. 1987. *The Power of Reason: 1988.* Washington, D.C.: Executive Intelligence Review.

Larson, Edward J. 1985. *Trial and Error: The American Controversy Over Creation and Evolution.* New York: Oxford University Press.

LaValley, Albert J. 1979. "The Stage and Film Children of Frankenstein: A Survey." In *The Endurance of Frankenstein: Essays on Mary Shelley's Novel,* ed. G. Levine and U. C. Knoepflmacher, 243–289. Berkeley and Los Angeles: University of Calif. Press.

Lawler, Donald. 1988. "Reframing Jekyll and Hyde: Robert Louis Stevenson and the Strange Case of Gothic Science Fiction." In *Dr. Jekyll and Mr. Hyde After One Hundred Years,* ed. W. Veeder and G. Hirsch, 247–261. Chicago: University of Chicago Press.

Lear, John. 1963. "The Real Danger in Fluoridated Water." *Saturday Review,* December 7:77–79.

———. 1964. "Documenting the Case Against Fluoridation." *Saturday Review,* January 4:85–92.

Levine, George. 1979. "The Ambiguous Heritage of Frankenstein." In *The Endurance of Frankenstein: Essays on Mary Shelley's Novel,* ed. G. Levine and U. C. Knoepflmacher, 3–30. Berkeley and Los Angeles: University of Calif. Press.

Lewenstein, Bruce V. 1995. "Do Public Electronic Bulletin Boards Help Create Scientific Knowledge? The Cold Fusion Case." *Science, Technology, and Human Values* 20:123–149.

Lincoln, Abraham. 1991. *Great Speeches.* New York: Dover.

McElheny, Victor E. 1985. "Impacts of Present-Day Popularization." In *Expository Science: Forms and Functions of Popularization,* ed. T. Shinn and R. Whitley, 277–282. Boston: Reidel.

McGraw, Onalee. 1976. "Secular Humanism and the Schools." Washington, D.C.: Heritage Foundation. Pamphlet.

McIverr, Thomas. 1989. "Creationism: Intellectual Origins, Cultural Context, and Theoretical Diversity." Ph.D. diss. University of California at Los Angeles.

Mallove, Eugene F. 1991. *Fire from Ice: Searching for the Truth Behind the Cold Fusion Furor.* New York: John Wiley and Sons.

Mander, Jerry. 1978. *Four Arguments for the Elimination of Television.* New York: Quill.

Mank, Gregory William. 1981. *It's Alive! The Classic Cinema Saga of Frankenstein.* San Diego: Barnes.

Margolis, Frederic J., and Sanford N. Cohen. 1985. "Successful and Unsuccessful Experiences in Combatting the Antifluoridationists." *Pediatrics* 76(1):113–118.

Marsden, George M. 1980. *Fundamentalism and American Culture.* Oxford: Oxford University Press.

———. 1989. "Evangelicals and the Scientific Culture." In *Religion and Twentieth-Century American Intellectual Life,* ed. M. J. Lacy, 23–48. Cambridge: Cambridge University Press.

Martin, Brian. 1988. "Analyzing the Fluoridation Controversy: Resources and Structures." *Social Studies of Science* 18:331 63.

———. 1989. "The Sociology of the Fluoridation Controversy: A Reexamination." *Sociological Quarterly* 30(1):59–76.

———. 1991. *Scientific Knowledge in Controversy: The Social Dynamics of the Fluoridation Debate.* Albany: State University of New York Press.

Marx, Leo. 1987. "Does Improved Technology Mean Progress?" *Technology Review,* January:33 ff.

Massey, Walter E. 1989. "Science Education in the United States: What the Scientific Community Can Do." *Science,* September 1, 245:915–921.

Mausner, Bernard, and Judith Mausner. 1955. "A Study of the Anti-Scientific Attitude." *Scientific American,* February:35–39.

Mayr, Ernst. 1978. "Evolution." *Scientific American,* September:47–55.

Mazur, Allan. 1973. "Disputes Among Experts." *Minerva,* 11:243–262.

———. 1981. "Media Controversies and Public Opinion on Scientific Controversies." *Journal of Communication* 31(2):106–115.

Mead, Margaret, and Rhoda Metraux. 1957. "Image of the Scientist Among High School Students." *Science,* 126:384 390.

Meier, Hugo A. 1957. "Technology and Democracy, 1800–1860." *Mississippi Valley Historical Review* 43:618–640.

Merton, Robert K. 1973a [1942]. "The Normative Structure of Science." In *The Sociology of Science: Theoretical and Empirical Investigations,* 267–278. Chicago: University of Chicago Press.

———. 1973b [1938]. "Science and the Social Order." In *The Sociology of Science: Theoretical and Empirical Investigations,* 254–266. Chicago: University of Chicago Press.

———. 1973c. *The Sociology of Science: Theoretical and Empirical Investigations.* Chicago: University of Chicago Press.

———. 1977. *The Sociology of Science: An Episodic Memoir.* Carbondale: Southern Illinois University Press.

Miller, Jon D. 1983. "Scientific Literacy: A Conceptual and Empirical Review." *Daedalus* 112(2):29–48.

———. 1987b. "The Scientifically Illiterate." *American Demographics,* June:26–31.

————. 1987a. "Scientific Literacy in the United States." In *Communicating Science to the Public,* ed. D. Evered and M. O'Connor, 19–37. New York: Wiley.

Morris, Henry M. 1963. *The Twilight of Evolution.* Grand Rapids, Mich.: Baker.

————. 1972. "Theistic Evolution." *Creation Research Society Quarterly* 8(4):271.

————. 1974. *The Troubled Waters of Evolution.* San Diego: Creation-Life.

————. 1982. "Evolution is Religion, Not Science." *Impact* (monthly mailing from ICR) 107.

————. 1983. "Creation Is the Foundation." *Impact* 126.

————. 1984. *A History of Modern Creationism.* San Diego: Master Books.

————. 1987. "Evolution and the New Age." *Impact* 165.

Morris, Henry M. and Duane Gish, eds. 1976. *The Battle for Creation.* San Diego: Creation-Life.

Morris, Henry M., Duane Gish, and George M. Hillestad, eds. 1974. *Creation: Acts, Facts, Impacts.* San Diego: Creation-Life.

Mueller, John E. 1968. "Fluoridation Attitude Change." *American Journal of Public Health* 58(10):1876–1882.

Mulkay, Michael. 1979. *Science and the Sociology of Knowledge.* London: George Allen and Unwin.

Murray, Edward. 1972. *The Cinematic Imagination.* New York: Frederick Ungar.

National Research Council. 1993. *Health Effects of Ingested Fluoride.* Washington, D.C.: National Academy Press.

NDPC (National Democratic Policy Committee). 1986. "A Vote for Proposition 64 Could Save the Life of Someone in Your Family." Washington, D.C.: National Democratic Policy Committee. Booklet.

Nelkin, Dorothy. 1982. *The Creation Controversy.* New York: Norton.

————. 1987. *Selling Science: How the Press Covers Science and Technology.* New York: Freeman.

Newell, Norman D. 1974. "Evolution Under Attack." *Natural History,* April:32–39.

Nitchie, Elizabeth. 1953. *Mary Shelley.* Westport, Conn.: Greenwood.

NOVA. 1990. *ConFusion in a Jar* (transcript of NOVA program of April 30, 1990). Boston, Mass.: BBC-TV and WGBH–Boston, for NOVA.

O'Brien, T. C. 1979. "Humanism, Christian." *Encyclopedic Dictionary of Religion.* Vol. F–N:1734. Washington, D.C.: Corpus.

Olson, Richard. 1975. *Scottish Philosophy and British Physics, 1750–1800.* Princeton: Princeton University Press.

Oppenheimer, G. M. 1988. "In the Eye of the Storm: The Epidemiological Construction of AIDS." In *AIDS: The Burden of History,* ed. E. Fee and D. M. Fox, 267–300. Berkeley and Los Angeles: University of Calif. Press.

OTGH (Old Time Gospel Hour). 1981. *Scientific Creation/Scientific Evolution Debate* (transcript of debate at Liberty Baptist College, October 13, 1981). Lynchburg, Va: Old Time Gospel Hour.

Paul, Benjamin D. 1959. "Synopsis of Report on Fluoridation." *Massachusetts Dental Society Journal* 8:19–21.

———. 1961. "Fluoridation and the Social Scientist: A Review." *Journal of Social Issues* 17(4):1–12.

Payer, Lynn. 1988. *Medicine and Culture.* New York: Penguin.

Peacock, James L. 1975. *Consciousness and Change.* Oxford: Basil Blackwell.

Peat, F. David 1989. *Cold Fusion: The Making of a Scientific Controversy.* Chicago: Contemporary Books.

Pfeiffenberger, Will, Ann Marie Zolandz, and Lee Jones. 1991. "Testing Physics Achievement: Trends Over Time and Place." *Physics Today,* September:30–37.

Piel, Gerard. 1986. "Natural Philosophy in the Constitution." *Science,* September 5, 233:1056–1060.

Pirie, David. 1973. *A Heritage of Horror: The English Gothic Cinema, 1946–1972.* London: Gordon Fraser.

Plaut, Thomas F. A. 1959. "Analysis of Voting Behavior in a Fluoridation Referendum." *Public Opinion Quarterly* 23(5):213–222.

———. 1960. "Practical Politics and Public Health." *Harvard Public Health Alumni Bulletin,* December:6–9.

Pollitzer, William S. 1980. "Evolution and Special Creation." *American Journal of Physical Anthropology* 53:329–330.

Pool, Robert.1989. "How Cold Fusion Happened—Twice!" *Science,* April 28, 244:420–423.

Popper, Karl. 1950. *The Open Society and Its Enemies.* Princeton: Princeton University Press.

Port, Otis. 1992. "Power in a Jar: The Debate Heats Up " *Business Week,* October 26:88–89.

Prawer, S. S. 1980. *Caligari's Children: The Film as a Tale of Horror.* Oxford: Oxford University Press.

Price, Don K. 1968 [1954]. "The Republican Revolution." In *The Politics of Science,* ed. W. R. Nelson, 5–25. New York: Oxford University Press.

ProFamily Forum. 1980. "Is Humanism Molesting Your Child?" Fort Worth, Tex.: ProFamily Forum. Pamphlet.

Rafferty, Max. 1969. "Guidelines for Moral Instruction in California Schools." Sacramento: California State Department of Education.

Rainie, Harrison, and Gary Cohen. 1991. "Congress's Most Feared Democrat." *U.S. News and World Report,* August 26:53–54.

Raman, Varadaraja V. 1975. "The Three Planes of Science in Society." *Impact of Science on Society* 25(1):9–17.

Reingold, Nathan. 1978. "O Pioneers!" *Wilson Quarterly* 2(3):55–64.

———. 1979. "Reflections on 200 Years of Science in the United States." In *The Sciences in the American Context,* ed. N. Reingold, 9–20. Washington, D.C.: Smithsonian Institution Press.

———. 1987. "Graduate School and Doctoral Degree: European Models and American Realities." In *Scientific Colonialism,* ed. N. Reingold and M. Rothenberg, 129–147. Washington, D.C.: Smithsonian.

Rodale, Robert. 1961. Letter to the editor. *Science,* September 22, 134:877–878.

Rosenberg, Charles E. 1966. "Science and American Social Thought." In *Science and Society in the United States,* ed. D. D. Van Tassel and M. G. Hall, 135–162. Homewood, Ill.: Dorsey.

Roush, Wade. 1992. "John Dingell: Dark Knight of Science." *Technology Review,* January:57–62.

Rousseau, Denis L. 1992. "Case Studies in Pathological Science." *American Scientist,* January–February, 80:54–63.

Rowland, F. Sherwood. 1993. "The Need for Scientific Communication with the Public." *Science,* June 11:260:1571–1576.

Rundall, Thomas G., and Kathryn A. Phillips. 1990. "Informing and Educating the Electorate About AIDS." *Medical Care Review* 47(1):3–13.

Rutherford, F. James. 1985. "Lessons from Five Countries." In *Science Education in Global Perspective,* ed. M. S. Klein and F. J. Rutherford, 207–231. Boulder, Colo.: Westview.

Sandeen, Ernest R. 1967. "Toward a Historical Interpretation of the Origins of Fundamentalism." *Church History* 36:66–83.

———. 1970. *The Roots of Fundamentalism.* Chicago: University of Chicago Press.

Sapolsky, Harvey M. 1968. "Science, Voters, and the Fluoridation Controversy." *Science,* October 25, 162:427–433.

Saposnik, Irving S. 1983. "The Anatomy of Dr. Jekyll and Mr. Hyde." In *The Definitive Dr. Jekyll and Mr. Hyde Companion,* ed. H. Geduld, 108–117. New York: Garland.

Scalia, Antonin. 1987. "Dissenting opinion in *Edwards* v. *Aguillard.*" *Law Week,* 55 LW 4860–4877.

Sclove, Richard E. 1994. "Citizen-Based Technology Assessment?" Amherst, Mass.: Loka Alert 1-12. Electronic.

———. 1995a. "Democratizing Science?" Amherst, Mass.: Loka Alert 2-3. Electronic.

———. 1995b. "Research for Communities." Amherst, Mass.: Loka Alert 2-5, Part 1. Electronic.

Scott, Pam, Evelleen Richards, and Brian Martin. 1990. "Captives of Controversy: The Myth of the Neutral Social Researcher in Contemporary Scientific Controversies." *Science, Technology, and Human Values* 15(4):474–494.

Seale, John R. 1984. "AIDS and Hepatitis B Cannot Be Venereal Diseases" (letter to the editor). *Canadian Medical Association Journal,* May 1, 130:1109–1110.

———. 1986. "Infectious AIDS" (letter to the editor). *Nature,* April 3, 320:391.

———. 1987a. "Kuru, AIDS, and Aberrant Social Behavior." *Journal of the Royal Society of Medicine,* April , 80:200–202.

———. 1987b. "Pathogenesis and Transmission of AIDS." *Veterinary Record* 120:454–59.

———. 1988. "Origins of the AIDS Viruses, HIV–1 and HIV–2: Fact or Fiction?" *Journal of the Royal Society of Medicine,* September, 81:537–539.

Segerstrale, Ullica. 1994. "Review of *The Golem,* by H. Collins and T. Pinch." *Science,* February 11, 263:837–838.

Shallis, Michael, and Philip Hills. 1975. "Young People's Image of the Scientist." *Impact of Science on Society* 25(4):275–278.

Shapin, Steven. 1982. "History of Science and its Sociological Reconstructions." *History of Science* 20:157–211.

———. 1993. "Mertonian Concessions." *Science,* February 5, 259:839–841.

Shaw, James H. 1954. "Should Fluorides Be Added to the Public Water Supplies?" *Scientific Monthly,* October, 79(4):232–240.

Shelley, Mary. 1964. *Frankenstein; or, the Modern Prometheus.* New York: Modern Library.

Shilts, Randy. 1988 [1987]. *And the Band Played On: Politics, People, and the AIDS Epidemic.* New York: Penguin.

Shortland, Michael. 1988. "Advocating Scientific Literacy and Public Understanding." *Impact of Science on Society* 38(4):305–316.

Simmel, Arnold, and David B. Ast. 1962. "Some Correlates of Opinion on Fluoridation." *American Journal of Public Health* 52(8):1269–1273.

Smith, Bruce L. 1991. "Scientism: The American Faith." *Minerva* 29(4):515–516.

Smith, Geoffrey E. 1988. "Fluoride and Fluoridation." *Social Science and Medicine* 26(4):451–462.

Sontag, Susan. 1966. "The Imagination of Disaster." In *Against Interpretation,* 209–225. New York: Farrar, Straus and Giroux.

Stevenson, Harold W. 1992. "Learning from Asian Schools." *Scientific American,* December:70–76.

Stevenson, Harold W., Chuansheng Chen, and Shin-Ying Lee. 1993. "Mathematics Achievement of Chinese, Japanese, and American Children: Ten Years Later." *Science,* January 1, 259:53–58.

Stevenson, Robert Louis. 1984. "The Strange Case of Dr. Jekyll and Mr. Hyde." In *Robert Louis Stevenson,* 643–687. London: Spring Books.

Storms, Edmund. 1994. "Warming up to Cold Fusion." *Technology Review,* May-June:19–29.

Taubes, Gary. 1993. *Bad Science: The Short Life and Weird Times of Cold Fusion.* New York: Random House.

———. 1995. "Epidemiology Faces Its Limits." *Science,* July 14, 269:164–69.

Tobey, R. C. 1971. *The American Ideology of National Science.* Pittsburgh: University of Pittsburgh Press.

Tocqueville, Alexis de. 1899 [1834]. *Democracy in America.* Vol. 2. New York: Appleton.

Toumey, Christopher P. 1990. "Sectarian Aspects of American Creationism." *International Journal of Moral and Social Studies* 5(2):116–142.

———. 1991. "Modern Creationism and Scientific Authority." *Social Studies of Science* 21(4):681–699.

———. 1992. "The Moral Character of Mad Scientists." *Science, Technology, and Human Values* 17(4):411–437.

———. 1993. "Evolution and Secular Humanism." *Journal of the American Academy of Religion* 61(2):275–301.

———. 1994. *God's Own Scientists: Creationists in a Secular World.* New Brunswick, N.J.: Rutgers University Press.

Traweek, Sharon. 1988. *Beamtimes and Lifetimes.* Cambridge, Mass.: Harvard University Press.

Webb, George E. 1983. "The 'Baconian' Origins of Scientific Creationism." *National Forum,* Spring, 63(2):33–35.

———. 1994. *The Evolution Controversy in America.* Lexington: University Press of Kentucky.

Whalen, Matthew D. 1981. "Science, the Public, and American Culture: A Preface to the Study of Popular Culture." *Journal of American Culture* 4(2):14–26.

White, W. H. Jr. 1956. *The Organization Man.* New York: Simon and Schuster.

Whitehead, John W., and John Conlan. 1978. "The Establishment of the Religion of Secular Humanism and Its First Amendment Implications." *Texas Tech Law Review* 10:1–66.

Whitley, Richard. 1985. "Knowledge Producers and Knowledge Acquirers." In *Expository Science: Forms and Functions of Popularization,* ed. T. Shinn and R. Whitley, 3–28. Boston: Reidel.

Wilstach, Paul. 1983. "Richard Mansfield and Jekyll and Hyde." In *The Definitive Dr. Jekyll and Mr. Hyde Companion,* ed. H. Geduld, 159–61. New York: Garland.

Winner, Langdon. 1986. *The Whale and the Reactor: A Search for Limits in an Age of High Technology.* Chicago: University of Chicago Press.

———. 1992. "Citizen Virtues in a Technological Order." *Inquiry* 35:341–61.

———. 1994. "The Mice That Roared." *Technology Review,* August-September:72

Wysong, R.L. 1976. *The Creation-Evolution Controversy.* Midland, Mich.: Inquiry Press.

INDEX

■ ■ ■

ABOUT THE AUTHOR

■ ■ ■

Christopher P. Toumey received his Ph.D. in anthropology at the University of North Carolina. He is the author of *God's Own Scientists* (Rutgers University Press, 1994), an ethnography of "scientific creationism," and of numerous articles on science. Currently he is working on his third book, a collection of stories about adventures in ethnography.